YOUR LIFE OR MINE

For Bina
Our two bodies, our one soul, are forever in love

and

In memory of my Grandmother
Jennie Bernstein
whose 1960 porcine heart valve gave her twenty more years
to share her kindness with the world

Your Life or Mine

How Geoethics Can Resolve the Conflict Between Public and Private Interests in Xenotransplantation

MARTINE ROTHBLATT, PhD
International Bar Association - United Therapeutics Corporation

ASHGATE

Published by
Ashgate Publishing Limited
Gower House
Croft Road
Aldershot
Hants GU11 3HR
England

Ashgate Publishing Company
Suite 420
101 Cherry Street
Burlington, VT 05401-4405
USA

Ashgate website: http://www.ashgate.com

British Library Cataloguing in Publication Data
Rothblatt, Martine, 1954-
Your life or mine : how geoethics can resolve the conflict between public and private interests in xenotransplantation
1.Xenografts - Moral and ethical aspects 2.Xenografts
3.Transplantation of organs, tissues, etc. - Complications
4.Zoonoses 5.Procurement of organs, tissues, etc. - Moral and ethical aspects 6.Procurement of organs, tissues, etc.
I.Title
174.2'4

Library of Congress Control Number: 2003112475

ISBN 0 7546 2391 2

Printed and bound in Great Britain by MPG Books Ltd, Bodmin, Cornwall

Contents

List of Tables and Figures

Preface

Organ transplantation extends life by replacing a failing organ with a graft from a recently deceased person or from a living donor. However, the supply of such replacement organs is much less than what is needed to extend the lives of most people with organ failure. Genetically-modified pig organs ("xenografts") and mechanical organs are the two most feasible ways of rectifying this shortage. This book focuses on the medical ethics of using xenografts to extend life in light of a public interest in minimizing the negative consequences of xenotransplantation.

Xenotransplantation presents a public health risk because new zoonoses can be introduced via the grafting of animal organs into humans. In addition, public opposition to xenotransplantation will arise if it is perceived as animal cruelty. Finally, xenotransplantation costs may clash with the public interest in optimal management of limited health care budgets. This book shows that each of these public interests can be resolved compatibly with xenotransplantation.

The xenograft recovery rules described fit within the societal consensus as to the fair treatment of pigs. Budgetarily speaking, at least a small number of xenotransplantation operations can be offered consistent with justice and health care rationing. The zoonotic disease risks of xenotransplantation can be acceptably contained with a three-prong strategy: (1) a ban on using graft sources other than herds believed to be pathogen-free; (2) a life-long, irrevocable commitment to bio-sampling by transplant recipients and their intimate contacts; and (3) a global program of random bio-sampling and basic health care to look for incipient new zoonoses. This book describes how the costs of this strategy can be funded with a tax on xenografts that is paid by the companies selling them. Risk allocation principles are shown to support a new regime of "geoethics" that mandates a global enforcement organization to assure consistency of private and public interests in xenotransplantation.

Acknowledgements

This book was a labor of love. It is largely based upon a Ph.D. thesis I completed in 2001. The taskmaster for that labor was Prof. Len Doyal. He devoted a great deal of time and effort analyzing with me whether I really understood what I thought I understood, and whether I really knew what I thought I knew. In true Socratic fashion, he let me see how very wrong I could be in my self-assessments. For that I am ever grateful. I cannot imagine that there could be a better thesis adviser than Prof. Doyal, for he put literally hundreds of hours into reading my drafts, and debating medical ethics with me. Into the future, my practice of Medical Ethics will always be, in large part, a reflection of the wisdom and reasoning that was imbued in me by Prof. Doyal.

Every good journey begins with an inspiration. My journey into Medical Ethics, as documented in this thesis, is true to form. The inspiration in this case came in part from my daughter Jenesis, and in part from Sir John Vane. Jenesis motivated me to seek out new cures for pulmonary diseases, and xenotransplantation holds great promise in that regard. Sir John encouraged me to pursue my quest, and introduced me to the Department of Human Science at Queen Mary College, St. Bartholomew and the Royal London School of Medicine and Dentistry.

I owe an enormous debt of gratitude to my brilliant friend and colleague, Teresa Bongartz. She challenged my thinking on a day-to-day basis and provided me with assistance in more ways than I can enumerate. She harnessed the power of the computer and the internet to help me find long-lost references, recover recently-lost thesis sections, and word process where no student has gone before. I cannot imagine any researcher being luckier than I simply because of my friendship with Ms. Bongartz.

I want to acknowledge the early training in speed-typing and library research provided to me by Rosa Lee Rothblatt. It never came in more handy than in working on this labor of love.

I am also most grateful for the flawless text management assistance of Robert Daye. In addition to his superb word processing skills, his cogent organization of my professional schedule was principally responsible for enabling me to find the time to complete this book.

Late in the final preparation of this book I had the good fortune to obtain the editing services of Rachel Turow. Her ideas, research and text editing resulted in a much improved book. I take responsibility for rebelliously insisting on the non-conforming use of "their" as a gender-neutral third-person plural substitute for the customary gender-specific third-person singular pronouns. There are undoubtedly many other errors that Ms. Turow did not have time to correct, and for which I claim ownership. For particularly well-parsed sentences, the reader should thank Ms. Turow, as do I.

Last but not least, I could never have succeeded without the unlimited moral support, culinary attention and loving patience offered by my soulmate, Bina Aspen Rothblatt. This book is the umpteenth example of the fact that, with you, all the good things in life are possible.

Chapter I

Introduction: The Organ Shortage is a Major Problem That Defies Conventional Solutions

Organ failure is a frequent cause of death. Human beings die when organs, such as the heart, lungs, liver, kidneys, pancreas or intestines, cease functioning. Heart disease is the biggest killer in North America and Europe. Approximately 750,000 people die each year of a failed heart in each continent ("Deaths," Table 17). Lung, liver and kidney disease are also major killers, due either to an organ-specific disease (such as pneumonia for the lungs), or to a cancer, which becomes lethal upon reaching the organ (such as skin cancer, which spreads to the liver). Assuming comparable populations and epidemiology, Europe and North America each suffer annual lung and liver or kidney tolls of approximately 120,000 and 50,000 lives respectively ("Deaths," Table 17). Summing up deaths due to organ failure in the North Atlantic region results in a body count of staggering proportions – about 210 people per hour.

The body is a kind of machine. If continued operation of a manufactured machine is desired, then it is necessary to replace key parts of such a machine prior to or upon its failure. Hence, it is possible to keep automobiles, aircraft and other manufactured machines operating indefinitely via periodic replacement of failing parts with newly manufactured spare parts. Society has now achieved the ability to extend the life of some people by replacing their failing organs. This science has remained immature because, unlike the potentially unlimited supply of mechanical spare parts, the human spare parts (organs) are harvested from a limited supply of dead people or, in the case of redundant organs (lungs, kidneys, liver sections), other, even more limited, living people. Furthermore, the harvested human organs rarely fit just right at the level of compatible biochemistry. The logistics of harvesting organs from the deceased, or from living donors, are vastly more problematic than the ordering of spare parts from a manufacturer's catalog. Consequently, it is easier to indefinitely extend the life of a jumbo jet than of a person.

Many people are working on the problem of how to regularize the availability of organs to extend human life. Ideas range from manufacturing organs out of synthetic materials (implantable "bio-machines"), to growing new organs from one's own differentiated cells (tissue engineering), to creating a global organ transplantation market (buying/selling human organs), to creating a supply of humanized organs grown within animals (xenotransplantation). As a result of these activities, the science of extending human life through organ transplantation will soon be as mature as the practice of extending the lives of complex mechanical machines.

The approach most likely to serve the most people in the next 10-20 years is that of xenotransplantation. However, this solution to extending human life is accompanied by a host of ethical and public policy issues centered around a conflict between private and public interests. It is to an analysis of these issues, and an assessment of the public/private conflict they engender, that this book is addressed.

Mind the Gap

An organ shortage first appeared in the mid-1980s when people who formally requested an organ began to have to wait increasingly lengthy (months, years) periods of time to get one. This organ shortage was due in part to the success of organ transplants, which attracted ever larger numbers of desperately hopeful patients. However, the organ shortage was also due to the increasing selectivity of transplant surgeons of the "quality" of organs they would accept for transplantation, since they saw firsthand that problematic organs resulted in poorer patient survival.

The organ shortage reached the public's consciousness by virtue of publicity about people who died awaiting transplant. However, the organ shortage is much worse than is generally acknowledged. Large numbers of people are screened out of the transplantation process before they have a chance to formally request an organ. And yet larger numbers of people are not even considered for transplantation because of *a priori* criteria established on the assumption of a severe organ shortage and other assumptions about equity, e.g., age, health, behavior, and social worth (Whitehead, p.481).

The organ shortage only appears to be a "small problem" amenable to tractable solutions such as increased voluntary organ donation. In fact, however, the organ shortage is a "large problem" that should be measured by the more than one million people who die each year due to the failure of a vital organ. Once the magnitude of this problem is frankly recognized, practical work on solutions can receive the priority they deserve.

Measurements of Demand and Supply

In the United States the United Network for Organ Sharing (UNOS) is responsible for measuring the demand and supply of organs. In the United Kingdom, the official responsibility for measuring organ demand and supply falls to the United Kingdom Transplant Support Service Authority (UKTSSA).

Beyond these two official sources of demand and supply measures, there is a robust literature of academic assessors of demand and supply. These scholarly experts generally believe that the demand for organs is significantly larger than admitted to by official sources. Also, it will be shown below, that were organ scarcity not a factor, the demand for organs would be orders of magnitude larger than today's official figures.

Demand for Hearts, Lungs, Livers and Kidneys

According to UNOS (UNOS, p.23), at the *end* of 1997 and *as of* May 6, 2000 the U.S. waiting list statistics (UNOS, p.23, *Transplant News*, p.2) for organs are:

Table I-1 Date-Specific Organ Wait List Totals

Organ	12/31/97	05/06/00
Hearts	3,899	4,159
Lungs	2,918	3,798 (Includes Heart/Lungs)
Livers	9,647	15,120
Kidneys	38,270	44,885

Another measure of demand is UNOS' report of the number of people who died while on the waiting list. That figure has remained quite constant in the 9 percent range each year, averaged over all organs (Buhler et al., p.416). However, excluding kidneys, for which dialysis is available as a bridge to transplantation, about 50 percent of the people on a waiting list die. Yet a third measure of demand is the wait times for an organ transplant. In the United States, these wait times can vary substantially by region, from an average of 96 days in the Southeast to 655 days in the Northeast (for livers) (Stolberg, p.A18).

Demand is also outstripping supply by growing amounts in the United Kingdom as well ("UK Donor," p.7). The waiting list for organs has grown to 5,500 persons in 2000 from 4000 persons in 1990, while only 1,400 kidney, 533 liver and 290 heart transplants were performed last year ("UK Donor," p.7). Most observers agree that the officially reported statistics dramatically underestimate the demand for organs. As the Nuffield Council on Bioethics observed:

> It is estimated that, if sufficient organs were available, the number of people in the UK who could benefit from heart transplantation would be five times the number that can currently hope to receive an organ. Since the incidence of heart failure increases with age, as the number of elderly people in the UK increases, the demand for heart transplants is likely to increase still further (Nuffield Council, p.4).

In the United States, officially stated demand understates actual demand due to the scarcity-induced medical screens described above for the UK and due to economic screening as a consequence of the profit-based U.S. health care system (Whitehead, p.481). A report by the prestigious Institute of Medicine observed that a "green screen" understates demand for organs because people who are unable to pay for an organ will generally not be added to the transplant wait list (Institute of Medicine 1996, p.65). Approximately 40.9 million, or 16 percent, of non-elderly Americans are uninsured (http://www.kff.org).

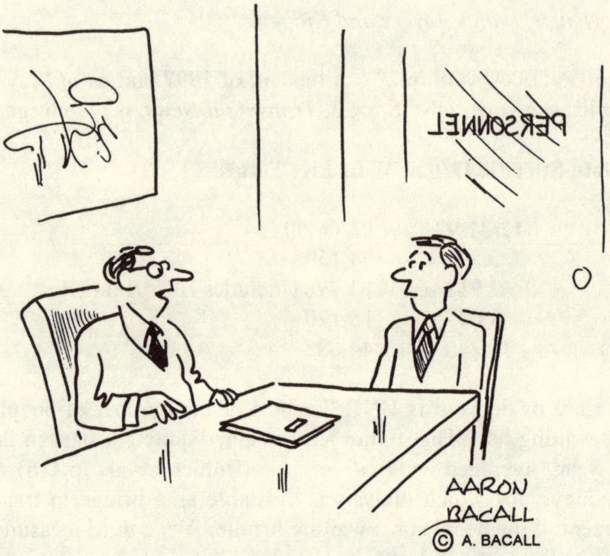

"We offer excellent medical coverage but the policy does not cover pre-existing organs."

Yet other observers quote far higher figures for latent demand for organ transplants (Evans, "Understanding," p.155). David Sachs, of Harvard Medical School, is one of the very few experts who have considered what the demand for organs might be in an era of abundance. He estimates that more than 400,000 people in the United States could annually benefit from heart transplants, compared to the current wait list of just over 4,000 persons ("Briefing," p.6665). A recently concluded study of the International Society for Heart and Lung Transplantation (ISHLT) notes that "the number of patients currently referred for HTx [Heart Transplantation] represents *only a small percentage* of those in whom transplantation (or some other form of cardiac replacements) could be considered" (Cooper et al. 2000, p.1147, emphasis added). Similarly, the ISHLT noted that official "Registry numbers *grossly underestimate* the potential demand for donor lungs because current age limits, organ shortage, and in many centers, other relative/absolute exclusionary criteria restrict programs from assessing the majority of people with end-stage lung failure" (Cooper 2000 et al., p.1152, emphasis added). The North American and European toll from vital organ failure is nearly 2 million persons a year. It would appear reasonable to estimate that a substantial number of these persons would be candidates for an organ transplant were scarcity not an issue (Cooper et al. 2000, p.1149).

In summary, the annual demand for organs ranges from low-end estimates provided by official agencies of thousands to tens of thousands for the UK and the US respectively to mid-range estimates five or more times as high to take account of drop-outs from the waiting list screening process. These estimates based on actual transplants or official waiting lists will be referred to as *extant demand*. But there are also high-end estimates based on other mortality and morbidity figures that might best be called *latent demand* – the demand for organs were they not scarce. These demand estimates would be in the range of a million organs a year for the US and Europe combined.

Historical, Current and Prospective Supply of Vital Organs

The history of supplying vital organs for transplantation is the story of how to get organs from those who would not miss them to those who are desperate to use them. The supply of organs is largely a function of the meaning of the phrase "would not miss them," a meaning that is constantly being redefined. The supply of organs is also, however, a function of new technology which continually expands the range of usable organs. An organ that is not wanted during one decade may very well, due to technological advances, be desperately desired ten years later. Constantly pushing the envelope of "who would not miss their organs" and "who is desperate to use them" has brought us to the present level of being able to save thousands of lives a year via transplantation. It has also brought us the dilemma of losing thousands of other lives due to an organ demand that outstrips supply. *This dilemma has now also brought us to the cusp of asking why not take the organs from animals? Will they miss them and can we use them?*

To start with, only "fresh" organs are wanted (Becker, p.216). Once a heart stops beating all of the body's vital organs rapidly (within minutes) lose their value as transplant organs – unless they are kept fresh in specially formulated cold solutions. The reason for this is that the cells and tissues that make up our vital organs rapidly begin to die and poison the organ without the supply of fresh oxygen obtained via continuously pumping blood from the heart. Hence the transplant community needed to find heart-beating donors that would not miss one or more of their organs. Such sources fell into the following categories:

- Living donors for one of a pair of redundant organs;
- Heart-beating, brain-dead donors for any organ.

Historically, the only living donors considered ethical to approach are, with very few exceptions, close relatives of a patient. The first such case occurred in 1954 when Dr. Joseph Murray performed the first successful kidney transplant in Boston (which helped earned him the Nobel Prize). This transplanted organ was not missed and could be used because it came from an identical twin brother. The brother willingly consented to the operation because only one of his two kidneys were needed for perfect health, he wanted to help his brother live, and the explanting process was not considered risky for the donor. As an identical twin, there was no risk of organ rejection, rendering the kidney useful in the pre-immunosuppressant 1950s.

Nine years later, with the benefit of Peter Medawar's insights into organ rejection and the first generation immunosuppressant azathioprine, Dr. Thomas Starzl was able to routinize kidney transplants at the University of Colorado for those persons with living related donors. However, the majority of those in need of a kidney transplant lacked an appropriate living related donor, and the marginal effectiveness of azathioprine kept demand for transplantation at a modest level. At that point the supply of donated organs was largely limited to living related donors, a source that still accounts for 25 percent of kidneys in the United States and 10 percent of kidneys in Europe (Ascher, p.394). Needless to say, such a source does not exist for hearts, and living related donation is still considered experimental for lungs and livers.

It was immediately obvious to people that the dead would not miss their organs, subject to religious concepts concerning post-death feelings. In the 1960s the vast majority of people considered someone dead when their heart stopped beating. Unfortunately, once a heart stops beating the body's vital organs rapidly become unusable for transplantation. Therefore, initial efforts at harvesting organs were focused on having a patient ready to be transplanted when and where another patient whose heart would soon stop beating was present. This approach produced very few successful transplants due to the logistical difficulties of matching deaths with recipients.

The disposition of dead people's bodies falls into two categories. Bodies that are dead due to accidents, homicides or suspicious circumstances are usually in the custody of a government agency (such as a Medical Examiner or Coroner) for a period of investigation. Bodies that are dead due to natural causes are the responsibility of their next of kin. The right to direct disposition of the body has been described in Canada as a "quasi-property" interest (Kennedy 1998, p.887), and the right to consent to medical uses of a corpse is often a subject of local (ordinance) legislation. Pioneering medical examiners were among the first to permit heart-beating, brain-dead bodies under their control to be used as a source of organs. However, throughout the 1960s, any surgeon who removed organs from a heart-beating patient risked being charged with homicide. Thus, a charade was often employed in which the heart-beating, brain-dead patient was prepared in an operating room for organ removal, but everything was placed on hold until natural processes actually caused a cessation of heartbeat. This provided relatively fresh organs, but was highly inefficient.

In 1967, in South Africa, Christiaan Barnard squarely faced the issue of transplanting from a non-heart-beating donor when he transplanted a heart from a brain-dead woman, Denise Darvall, into heart-failure patient Louis Washkansky. Bernard argued that the brain-dead woman was dead, and there was no point in waiting for the heart to stop beating to confirm that fact. (In fact, the donor heart was asystolic at the actual time of transplantation). Almost overnight, everyone saw that acceptance of brain death as death was the best way to obtain transplantable hearts, and to thereby save the lives of others.

In August 1968, Harvard's Ad-Hoc Committee on Irreversible Coma published standards of brain death in the *Journal of the American Medical Association*. The Harvard publication clearly stated that a person was dead when the brain death criteria were met; there was no need to wait for the heart to stop beating. By 1970, nearly every U.S. State had codified the brain death criteria. The class of people who now would not "miss their organs" included heart-beating, brain-dead persons, subject to the consent of those entitled to the bodies. This greatly expanded the *useable* supply of vital organs. Instead of recovering useable organs only from bodies whose hearts stopped in the hospital, it was now possible to also recover organs from bodies, usually trauma victims, whose brains died outside the hospital and were still heart-beating upon arrival.

It is generally agreed that the high-powered immunosuppressor cyclosporine, first made available in the late 1970s, is the single most important factor in causing organ demand to surge in excess of supply (Porter, p.619). Cyclosporine enabled much greater long-term survival success than its weaker predecessor immunosuppressives, and simultaneously eliminated much of the mortality differences between donated organs from genetically linked relatives or cadaveric strangers. Many more physicians now felt it reasonable to refer end-stage patients to transplant centers; indeed, for many conditions transplantation became a "standard of care" option. Surging demand served as the impetus for new organizations to be formed that specialized in supplying organs.

Organ procurement organizations were formed soon thereafter to "harvest" organs from the brain-dead, heart-beating persons. These organizations accomplish their task by educating the public of the need for them to make known the desire to donate their organs, by persuading relatives to donate their deceased family member's organs, by persuading medical examiners to donate the organs of brain-dead, heart-beating bodies in their possession, and by ensuring that local hospitals facilitate the organ donation process.

The results of organ procurement efforts have been to achieve a level of cadaveric organ donation that has grown in the United States from 10,794 organs from 4,083 donors in 1988, to 14,734 organs from 4,859 donors in 1993, to 16,244 organs from 5,475 donors in 1997 (Johnson, p.52, UNOS, p.1). In addition, living donors have increased from 1,824 in 1988 to 3,793 in 1997, almost all of which are donations of a single kidney. Expressed in terms of donations per million population, the 1997 figure represents approximately 20 donors per million and 60 organs per million. It is clear that the rate of increase in organ donation from 1993 to 1997 is much less than from 1988 to 1993. The UNOS website, http://www.unos.org, provides data through 2001 which is little different from the published data provided above: 17,279 organs from 5,843 cadaveric donors plus 4,662 living donors. In short, organ donation is flat over the past several years. For example, there were only sixteen more donors in 2000 than in 1999 (*Transplant News*, p.1).

By comparison, at the West's approximate 0.9 percent annual death rate ("Deaths," Table 17), 9,000 people per million die each year, the vast majority of whom are considered too old or too diseased to donate organs, and who are also excluded from receiving organs via transplant screening criteria. If any appreciable percentage of the annual death rate were to be blunted with organ transplantation, it is clear that a vast increase in donated organs would be necessary. For example, out of the West's 9,000 per million annual death rate, approximately 3,000 people per million die of heart failure, 400 people per million die of non-infectious lung disease and 200 people per million die of non-malignant liver or kidney disease ("Deaths," Table 17). Hence, even if two kidneys and a liver were taken from each organ donor, the U.S. organ donor rate of 20 donors per million would save only 60 people per million out of the 200 people per million who die from liver or kidney disease. Cadaveric organ donation falls still further behind in terms of needed lung transplants (40 lungs per million assuming one lung goes to each of two recipients compared to 400 people per million dying of lung disease). Cadaveric heart availability falls short of even 1 percent of the number of needed hearts to combat deaths due to heart disease (which conservatively excludes deaths due to "cardiovascular diseases" such as artherosclerosis and stroke, much of which could be delayed with a new heart).

In the United Kingdom, the level of organ donors has remained nearly steady since 1990, at about 1000 persons per year, or slightly below the US level in terms of donors per million (Nuffield Council, p.16). Relatives in the UK refuse organ donation about 30 percent of the time, above the US refusal rate of 23 percent (Nuffield Council, p.15). Since the supply of organs is much less than 30 percent below the demand for organs, however, it is clear that increased organ donation alone cannot satisfy transplant organ demand. Indeed, the current UK "donor identity plan" is expected to increase heart and liver transplants by only 10 percent ("UK Donor," p.7). This is far below the 500 percent increase called for by the Nuffield Council (Nuffield Council, p.4). Elsewhere in Europe organ donor rates range from 25 per million in Austria (yielding 87 organs per million) to 10 per million in the Netherlands (yielding 31 organs per million) (*Transplant News*, May 14, 2000, p.1). As with elsewhere, these organ donation rates are well below the death rates attributable to organ failure. Brazil performed 3,500 organ transplants in 2000 ("Brazil," p.6). India performed 3,000, mostly kidney transplants in the same year, as compared to 89,000 new cases of chronic renal failure that present annually ("Huge," p.7).

Where Have All the Organs Gone?

It will be a challenge for current or prospective organ procurement initiatives to significantly close the organ shortage gap. As shown below, nearly half of all cadaveric organs are simply deemed unsuitable:

Table I-2 Heart-Beating, Brain-Dead Potential Donors in the U.S.

(n = 66 approached donors per million)

Unsuitable (e.g. infectious disease present)	47%
Consented to Donation	30%
Consent Refused	23%

(General Accounting Office, p.10)

Hence, even if consent to donation was no longer a problem, cadaveric organ transplantation rates would not exceed 35 per million persons – enough to cover 50 percent of the latent demand for kidneys and livers (assuming three organs per decedent), 18 percent of the latent demand for lungs (assuming two lungs per decedent), and less than 2 percent of the latent demand for hearts.

There are at least five initiatives underway that could prospectively increase the number of donor organs available. One purpose of these initiatives is to reach beyond the current brain-dead, heartbeating donors to a larger pool of candidates. For example, in the United States there are 75,000 car accident, suicide and homicide victims annually, a rate of 300 persons per million. Similarly, even with automobile fatalities down 26 percent from 1990, some 43,000 people died in European road accidents during 1998, a fatality rate of 114 persons per million (with a range from Sweden's 60 road deaths per million to Portugal's 243 road deaths per million) ("EU Road," p.2). It can therefore be clearly seen from the statistics given above that there is room for more organs to be harvested.

Five organ procurement initiatives that aim to expand the pool of harvested organs are: (1) presumed consent, (2) use of organs from persons in a persistent vegetative state, (3) use of organs from elective ventilated donors, (4) use of organs from non-heart-beating donors, and (5) revisions to allocation criteria and improved infrastructure.

Presumed Consent

In most countries, an organ may be removed for transplantation only after the donor or their next of kin has so consented. However, in a few countries, laws have been implemented that presume consent to organ donation upon death, unless an objection has been registered. This presumed consent is also known as "opting out" or "contracting out." Four western countries have adopted this kind of a system in the hope of increasing organ donation: Brazil, Spain, Austria and Belgium. It has been difficult to assess unambiguously whether or not presumed consent increases organ donation because studies have been confounded with other factors that affect organ donation rates. These confounding factors include improved organ procurement training and better hospital infrastructure on the one hand, and falling numbers of road accidents on the other. Equally, even in circumstances where donor consent is explicit, transplant teams are loathe to use organs in the face of family objections. Nevertheless, there is evidence from Belgium that presumed consent increases donation substantially – by 160 percent in only three years (Kennedy and Grubb 2000, p.1650). However others dispute the accuracy of the correlation between high post-mortem removal rates and presumed consent laws (Ascher, p.393).

An additional benefit attributed to presumed consent is that it relieves an emotional burden to the family of having to make an organ donation decision. Even though the decision could still be available to families, the weight of the decision would be lightened by knowing that the deceased never decided to "opt out" of presumed consent, and thus would have agreed with organ donation. In Belgium, less than 2 percent of the population opts out of presumed consent and families, when asked, object only 10 percent of the time as compared to 20-30 percent of the time in other European countries (Kennedy and Grubb 2000, p.1651). Notwithstanding the apparent benefits of presumed consent, Germany, the UK and all American States have steadfastly refused to use it.

The reluctance of so many countries to implement presumed consent is morally troubling. Rarely are there situations in which the moral reasons (save lives) to do an act (harvest organs from cadavers) are so strong as compared to the reasons to forebear (avoid impinging upon the superstitions of decedents or their families). John Harris, one of England's leading bioethicists, rightly proposes that we clear the medico-legal decks here by declaring cadavers the property of the State:

> Indeed it seems clear that the benefits from cadaver transplants are so great, and the reasons for objecting so transparently selfish or superstitious, that we should remove altogether the habit of seeking the consent of either the deceased or relatives. This we already do when post-mortem examinations are ordered without any consents being required and despite the fact that these too involve interference with the dignity of a dead body and the removal (albeit temporarily) of organs. It has always seemed to me curious that the state can order a post-mortem examination to satisfy its curiosity about the cause of death, but not order cadaver transplants in order to save the lives of living citizens (Harris, *Clones*, p.125).

Based on the above-described statistics from Belgium with presumed consent, Harris' proposal can be expected to more than double the supply of organs. While such an increase in organ supply will make an important difference to many patients, it will still fall far short of meeting the latent demand for organs.

Permanent Vegetative State (PVS)

Another prospective source of donor organs is from persons in a PVS, including possibly anencephalic neonates (persons born with only the stem portion of their brain). There are an estimated 10,000-25,000 adult US patients, 4,000-10,000 child US patients and 1,000 UK patients in a PVS (Hoffenberg, p.1320). Additionally, about 1,000 anencephalic infants are born each year. Assuming correct diagnosis, none of these individuals has any chance of sentient life (they lack higher brain function). It is also the case that none of them are wholly "brain-dead" (they retain brain stem activity). Would they miss their organs and would they be useful?

Currently, organs may not be used from PVS and anencephalic individuals until they have died a natural death or have had death induced through withdrawal of fluids and nutrients. Unfortunately, at that point the organs are rarely of any utility because the individuals have by then been starved of nutrients or suffered multiple organ failure. Therefore, one prospective means of increasing the supply of organs is to cause a prompt death of these individuals by the removal of their organs for transplantation, or by other means while keeping their organs transplantable. It has been argued that this would not harm the PVS or anencephalic individuals if it were done only as an alternative to removal of feeding, since it is presumed in that case that the individual feels no pain and lacks sentience (Hoffenberg, p.1321). As an additional benefit, the family and caregivers would be relieved of the pain of seeing a slow deterioration, and would be buoyed by the knowledge that at least a "gift of life" was made via organ donation.

Prior to PVS and anencephalic patients becoming a source of donated organs, there will have to be legal changes either to the definition of brain death or to exempt such patients from legal prohibitions against killing. The current definition of brain death requires irreversible cessation of all functions of the entire brain, including the brain stem (Culpepper, p.28). This definition could be modified to require irreversible cessation of higher brain function only, perhaps for a specified period of time such as several months or a year. However, notwithstanding a 1995 decision of the Council on Ethical and Judicial Affairs of the American Medical Association that it is ethically acceptable to use brain-stem living anencephalic infants as organ donors, in no place in America is such a practice allowed (Council on Ethical and Judicial Affairs, p.581). The prospects may be even less hopeful for using PVS donors to increase the supply of organs since, on rare occasions, inaccurately diagnosed PVS patients do in fact recover. Opponents of using PVS patients for organ donors are sure to use this fact to strengthen their case.

Elective Ventilated Donors

One of the current efforts to increase the supply of donated organs involves the use of an elective ventilation protocol. In essence, this approach is just one more effort to expand the scope of "unmissed" yet useful organs. Elective ventilation is a procedure for keeping a person's lungs operating, and their heart beating (the heart stops beating within minutes of oxygen deprivation), after a decision has been made that the person is certain to die – although that person has not yet satisfied the criteria set for whole-brain death. For example, persons who suffer a severe brain trauma or hemorrhage will usually die. In some such cases the death proceeds first by loss of higher brain function, then loss of respiration, then loss of heartbeat and finally loss of brainstem function. Only after the last loss, however, is the patient considered brain-dead. At that point the utility of the person's organs for transplantation will have deteriorated. The idea behind elective ventilation is to keep the person's lungs (and hence heart) working after they fail and until there is loss of brain stem activity. Once full-brain death can be declared, then the organs can be transplanted in optimal form since they will be "heart-beating donor" organs, the freshest kind.

The use of elective ventilation is controversial. The practice has been barred in England and Wales because it is considered an unlawful battery (Price, p.170). The logic for opposition to the procedure is based on the observation that *perforce* the patient is not yet dead or else their organs would have been taken immediately. Consequently, since the patient is not yet dead, and since there is no therapeutic (to the patient) reason for the elective ventilation, it must be an infringement upon that person's bodily integrity, i.e., a battery.

The opposition to elective ventilation may yet fall to the logical argument that it is only our ability to measure death, or our willingness to declare it, that makes the patient alive; that in fact elective ventilation is simply causing the perfusion of a body that is devoid of higher brain function. Once we are willing to concede that an irreversible cessation of heart and lung function, coupled with higher brain death, constitutes death, then there should not be further objection to the use of elective ventilation. For the moment, however, the continuation of heart-lung function by artificial means is proscribed as a method of increasing the supply of heart-beating donors.

Non-Heart-Beating Donors

The use of non-heart-beating donors has been called "back to the future" because it is with these kinds of organs that transplantation began. Prior to the acceptance of "brain-death" in the late 1960s, organs could only be taken from non-heart-beating donors because only those bodies were deemed dead. However non-heart-beating donor organs always present a "warm ischemia" problem – specifically, the longer an organ has been without blood supply (ischemia) and warm, the worse it functions after being transplanted. Consequently, once brain-death was accepted, transplant surgeons demanded organs only from heart-beating donors since those organs had minimal warm ischemia (they are perfused with blood until explanted, then immediately placed in a special cold transplant solution for transport, and then rapidly reperfused upon transplantation). The surgeons' preference was backed by studies showing significantly better transplantation success rates with heart-beating donors as compared to non-heart-beating donors (Eckhoff, p.187).

The worsening organ shortage has spurred a reexamination of the utility of non-heart-beating donor organs. The reexamination is also being nurtured by published studies from Japan (which has yet to fully embrace brain-death) showing good results with whole-body cooling immediately upon declaration of death. This reduces the "warmth" aspect of unwanted warm ischemia. Studies at the University of Wisconsin showed an 8.6 percent increase in organs transplanted by their center as a consequence of accepting non-heart-beating organs. An even more aggressive program, which uses non-heart-beating organs from "uncontrolled environments," such as highway accidents, as well as "controlled environments," such as hospitals, yielded a 20 percent increase in transplantable organs (Kootsra et al., p.910). New techniques are being tested which perfuse (via cannula) non-heart-beating donor organs with special solutions prior to their explantation to enable them to better withstand warm ischemia. Ultimately, a substantial number of accidental deaths could give rise to organ donation regardless of whether the donors are heart-beating.

Originally it was believed that the annual donor pool was approximately 100 donors per million (Bollinger and Salvatierra, p.411), compared to an automobile accident death rate of nearly 150 persons per million. Rates today are only about 20-25 donors per million (Ascher, p.390). Part of the shortfall from the 100 donor per million target population is due to reticence in using non-heart-beating or other problematic donors, and the rest is due to donor refusal. Even if the entire donor pool were successfully accessed, however, the number of donated hearts would still fall far short of the heart failure death rate of 3,000 persons per million (American Medical Association, p.768). Indeed, organ supplies would have to be more than three times current levels to even satisfy the liver and kidney failure death rate of 200 persons per million. Clearly then, historical, current and prospective supplies of vital organs from human donors *will not* solve humanity's need for replacement parts.

Improved Allocation and Infrastructure

With new donor supplies clearly limited, it is logical to ask if the organ gap could be closed through better management of those organs that are available. For example, if organs were allocated to only those most at risk of dying, would all demand be satisfied by conserving organs for only the sickest, not those with the greatest potential for life. Or, vice versa, could the greatest number of life years be achieved by only giving organs to those with the greatest chance of surviving? Similarly, if organ procurement and transplantation infrastructure were improved, would a larger percentage of available organs be used rather than lost to "warm ischemia?" If organ transplant counselors were better trained, would more living relatives be asked and agree to offer their own redundant organs for transplant to family members in need? If surgeons were better trained, would living related lung and liver donations become as common as living related kidney donations?

Waiting lists for organs are prioritized according to a set of criteria. The two main factors that move people up the list are the amount of time they have been on the list and the imminence of their predicted death. Other relevant factors include their location and their compatibility factors, such as blood type. The waiting list criteria are different for each kind of organ due to organ-unique factors affecting the success of transplantation. The waiting list criteria are drawn up by experts who seek to balance conflicting interests of fairness to patients, encouragement of organ donation, and maximization of successful outcome. As might be expected for any such system, when people's lives are at stake, there are perennial arguments as to whether or not any set of criteria is making the best use of available organs.

It is highly doubtful that any reprioritization of waiting list criteria would have a major impact on the organ shortage. For example there is a current dispute in the United States over whether livers should go first to the sickest people nationwide (new system, under legal challenge) or be offered first to those with compatible blood factors locally, and only if there are no matches, then to regional and national waiting lists (previous system). The proponents of a change argue that, at most, 200 additional lives would be saved each year (Stolberg, p.A18). This is clearly significant, but still only a step toward alleviating the 1000 per year liver waiting list deaths (Stapleton, p.11). And opponents of the change dispute that any benefit will result at all due to higher organ failure rates in the most seriously ill (Stolberg, p.A18). In the words of bioethicist Arthur Caplan, "It's as if we were in a lifeboat and instead of trying to figure out how many of us might survive a shortage of food and water, we said 'let's pick the people who are closest to dead and save them'" (Stolberg, p.A18). In any event, as a point of reference, the total annual liver disease death toll approaches 100 persons per million, or about 25,000 persons annually in the United States (American Medical Association, p.768). Hence, much more than different allocation procedures will be needed to address the real organ shortage. Indeed, critics claim that changing the allocation procedures merely changes the postal codes of those who die (McMullen, p.423).

Aside from allocation criteria, improvements in transplantation infrastructure are another path to closing the organ gap. These improvements may be as basic as increasing the number of intensive care beds, because if patients are not dying in the hospital then it is much more difficult to obtain useable organs. But in today's era of health care cost containment, the trend is toward keeping patients out of the hospital as much as possible. Consequently, infrastructure improvements may not be a realistic means of reducing the organ gap.

Alternatively, investments may be made in transplantation outreach services. Modest investments in equipping and training ambulance teams for minimizing warm ischemia has been shown to increase organ procurement by up to 20 percent in the Maastricht region of Holland. Fielding better trained organ procurement coordinators would also likely result in enhanced organ donation rates. However, as mentioned earlier, these improvements will occur at the margin since, already, half the organs are rejected as unusable and relative rejections, even if totally eliminated, would only double the number of organs made available. While this would be a huge improvement for those currently on organ transplantation waiting lists, it would do little to handle the latent demand for organ transplants likely to materialize en masse if the waiting lists ever shrunk.

A final infrastructure-type improvement could have a truly major impact upon organ availability for kidneys, livers and lungs – an increase in the use of organs from living related donors. Most people in need of a transplant have a relative with a spare kidney, regenerable liver lobe or explantable lung lobe. Were all these relatives willing to part with the spare organ or organ segment, waiting lists would exist only for hearts. Unfortunately, this is not the case. While an admirable 25 percent of U.S. kidney transplants are from living related donors, only 10 percent of Europeans volunteer a kidney to a relative (Ascher, p. 394). And today, only a miniscule percentage of livers and lungs are transplanted from living donors (Callender, p.347).

The liver is an especially remarkable organ in that it re-grows to its full size in both the donor and the recipient after the smaller of its two segments is transplanted (Scott, p.156). Unfortunately, the operation is grueling, taking as many as 12 hours and the informed consent process appears to frighten most relatives away – or at least tends to make all parties rely first on the transplant list. Nevertheless, there seems to be little reason why living related liver transplantation could not, in theory, largely eliminate liver waiting list problems. In addition, for those fulminant liver failure patients whose livers are still capable of regeneration, the temporary use of an external liver-support device for a few days or weeks while their own liver regenerates can avoid the need for a liver transplant (Abouna 2001, p.123).

Each of our two lungs consists of three lobes. A series of operations at leading U.S. hospitals have demonstrated the feasibility of transplanting one or two lobes from a parent to a child with outcomes equal or better to those achieved with cadaveric lungs. Both the donor and recipient suffered no diminution in their quality of life, notwithstanding a smaller lung volume (Ascher, p.405).

Finally, a small number of partial pancreas transplants among family members have demonstrated the feasibility of this kind of living related donor procedure. The donor and recipient each end up with half a pancreas (Ascher, p.400). While their laboratory results betray a diminished level of pancreatic functionality, this does not appear to affect their well-being.

One of the reasons given for lack of a greater number of living related donor procedures is that transplant coordinators fear subtle coercion of the relative (Ascher, p.394). Such coercion would violate the bioethical principle of informed consent. For different reasons, though, transplantation officials discourage organ donations from unrelated parties unless there is an emotional bond with the recipient. In particular, organ donations will be disallowed if there is any sign of a commercial relationship or non-altruistic motive (*Transplant News*, August 12, 2000, p.4).

Given the singular potential of living organ donations to alleviate extant – and even latent – organ shortages, it is incumbent upon us to next explore whether economic incentives are, in fact, contra-ethical. Most scarce things in life are allocated by economics. Will we soon have a marketplace solution for the organ shortage problem as well?

Selling Your Body: The Status of Marketplace Solutions to the Problem

The general concept of marketplace solutions to the demand for humans, or pieces of them, is as old as slavery. One reason certain slaves, such as gladiators, were purchased was to gain courage by drinking their blood. Similarly, ancient Egyptian royalty bathed in blood "to refresh their powers" (Titmuss, p.61). People have sold their hair and teeth for centuries (Hugo, pp.185-86). By 1910, commercial sales of mothers' breastmilk were netting crews of women in Boston, Massachusetts $4.20 per week (Weaver and Williams, p.324). Commercial sales of blood remain a big business in many countries throughout the world, including the US and India.

Vital organs are not like blood or breastmilk. Major surgery is needed to remove a vital organ for transplantation. This surgery is considered minimally risky for the removal of kidneys (sixteen reported living donor deaths out of tens of thousands of procedures), and somewhat risky for the removal of a portion of the liver, pancreas or lungs (one living donor death out of less than a hundred procedures). Nevertheless, aside from the surgical risk, an otherwise healthy person donating a kidney, liver section, pancreas segment or lung lobe is not considered to have reduced their lifespan or quality of life. Hence the question naturally arises: why should people not be allowed to sell parts of their body to help redress the organ shortage?

People are allowed to risk their lives in work and recreational activities. Why not permit people to take a small risk of death in order potentially to save the lives of recipients, while being compensated?

In fact, nowhere in the world is it legal to buy or sell any vital organ (*Transplant News*, February 29, 2000, p.5). This is a somewhat surprising situation in light of humanity's long history of commerce in people and some of their tissues or fluids. The global ban on commerce in vital organs – implemented via national legislation in most countries and medical practice norms everywhere – arises from three separate bases:

- The organ procurement establishment believes that the total number of transplantable organs will go down if people can sell their organs because more people will cease donating their organs than will begin selling their organs. The supply side logic here is that any financial incentives for donating organs will sharply undermine a fragile and as yet incomplete public consensus that looks at cadaveric organ donation as a social duty – a consensus that took thirty years to develop. The organ procurement establishment also opposes organ sales based on historical evidence that sold blood is more likely to be tainted with viruses than is voluntarily donated blood. They fear that organs bought from desperate people will be more likely to be diseased, and could thus spread disease the way purchased blood spread hepatitis.

- Nearly all opinion leaders in the field of bioethics and health policy believe that organ sales are wrong for reasons based on lack of consent due to financial duress and on loss of human dignity and social solidarity as a consequence of "commodification of body parts." These opinion leaders believe a benevolent paternalism is necessary to protect people from selling their own body parts.[1]
- There is overwhelming public revulsion at the concept of buying and selling vital organ parts. The reasons given for this revulsion generally include strong feelings about taking advantage of large disparities in wealth or about any kind of cannibalization of people.

Notwithstanding the universal official stand against an organ market, a few brave souls have presented counter-arguments in favor of a trade in body parts. It is important to consider each of these counter-arguments because of the possibility that an organ market could satisfy much or conceivably all of the demand for

---

[1] The courts are reluctant to recognize a property right in body parts, as was exemplified by the decision in *Moore v. Regents of University of California*. *Moore v. Regents of University of California, 51 Cal. 3d 120 (1991).* Moore's cells were used for medical research in order to start a cell line that was used to develop drugs to treat a form of leukemia. At the time of the removal of the cells, Moore was unaware of the use to which they would be put. Moore argued that the use of his cells in this way without his consent constituted conversion and that he was entitled to some of the revenue from the sale of the cell line. The court held that the use of Moore's cells for medical research was not conversion. Patients have no right of ownership once their cells have left their bodies. Informed consent laws are adequate to protect patients from abuse by their physicians. The court was also especially concerned that imbuing body parts with a property right would dampen medical research. This legal controversy has been further extended to gametes. It is especially interesting to consider the use of sperm that has been extracted from a newly dead husband in order that his widow might still bear his child. See, for example, Lori B. Andrews, *The Body, Economic Power and Social Control*, 75 Chi.- Kent L. Rev. 3 (1999); Andrews, *Alternative Reproduction*, S. Cal. L. Rev. 623 (1991); Andrews, *The Gene Patent Dilemma: Balancing Commercial Incentives With Health Needs*, 2002 Hous. J. Health L. & Pol'y 65 (2002).

organs. For example, the number of people living with an explantable kidney, liver segment or lung lobe vastly surpasses the number of people who die each year due to kidney, liver or lung diseases. Were there a way to persuade healthy people to donate these organs to strangers, even the latent organ shortage would be solved. With regard to hearts, the ability to enter into futures contracts to sell one's heart upon death might, within a couple decades, produce a large enough supply of hearts to satisfy at least a modest multiple of the current waiting list demand for hearts.

Supply Side Economics Justification for Banning Organ Sales

The organ procurement establishment consists of professionals responsible for creating a supply of transplantable organs for surgeons and their hospitals. The virtually unanimous view of these individuals is that legalizing the buying and selling of organs from donors would result in fewer transplantable organs. This contradicts traditional economic theory since the supply of a good usually increases with the price paid for it. If no price is paid, then the supply will remain fixed at a level obtainable via exhortations to donate the good. However, if the people making donations see that others are making money from offering the same good, then it is logical to conclude that the people making donations will demand like compensation, or will cease making donations.

For example, 40 percent of New Zealand blood donors in a survey said they would no longer give blood "if profits were to be made from selling blood products" (Howden-Chapman et al., p.1131). Perhaps more to the point, Richard Titmuss' classic study of blood supply discovered that while the rate of paid blood donations in New York rose from 15 percent in 1952 to 55 percent in 1966, the proportion of voluntary donations fell from 20 percent in 1956 to about 1 percent in 1966 (Titmuss, p.152). This quantitative analysis could not be extrapolated generally due to poor reporting among U.S. blood banks and a plethora of not-voluntary and not-paid donors, such as those donating as part of union activities or those who received non-cash benefits.

These supply side economic justifications for banning a trade in organs are vulnerable to criticism. First, fewer voluntary donations do not translate, *ipso facto*, into fewer donations overall. It may well be that total donations (of blood or organs) increase in a market-based system, as economic theory would predict, because new suppliers exceed those turned off by commercialism. In *The Gift Relationship*, Titmuss tried, but could not, demonstrate that total U.S. blood donations fell as the country shifted from a voluntary to a market-oriented system. He was, however, able to convincingly demonstrate that, at least in the 1950s and 1960s, a market-based system entailed substantially higher per-unit costs for blood and inferior blood quality as measured by higher rates of blood-borne pathogens. (There are poorly substantiated allegations that voluntary donations dropped soon after paid donations of blood were permitted in certain places) (Gore, p.290).

The findings of Titmuss do not lend much support to supply side arguments against a trade in organs. Even if purchased organs are more expensive than donated organs, that is a price many would be willing to pay when the alternative is death. This is different in the case of blood, where there was simply a replacement of free blood with paid blood. In the organ arena, there is a replacement of no organs with paid organs.

The cost-differential is further mooted by the facts that American hospitals apply a huge profit mark-up to procured organs, surgeons get large sums for their transplantation handiwork, and the organ procurement organizations themselves charge thousands of dollars for "harvesting" the organs from grieving families' decedents and transporting them nationwide. Indeed, nearly everyone in the organ transplantation "loop" appears to profit from the process except the donor. Purchased organs, with scheduled explant surgeries perhaps in the same hospital as the transplant, may in fact be less expensive than paying organ procurement organizations to harvest organs under roadway death conditions and ship them nationwide. Blood banking technologies – and efficiencies – are quite different from those pertinent to organ procurement.

Regarding pathogenic pollution of purchased tissues, government regulations can (but did not in the 1950s and 1960s) require equally rigorous testing of paid and voluntary suppliers. Certainly one lesson learned from the AIDS tragedy is that all bodily fluids, from every body, must be considered infectious until proven otherwise. The American Medical Association has observed, in expressing limited support for modest financial payments to an estate if the decedent agreed when alive to post-mortem harvesting of their organs:

> In recent years, routine donor and laboratory screening tests have largely eradicated any quality differences between blood plasma from unpaid vs. paid donors. In addition, in one recent study, paid cytapheresis donors were shown to be just as safe as unpaid whole blood donors when donors were subjected to adequate screening on the basis of laboratory tests and assessment of high-risk behaviors (Council on Ethical and Judicial Affairs, p.586).

Even in the face of these arguments, defenders of a market ban still counter-argue that conventional economics "depends on critical assumptions which are especially unrealistic in the case of organ procurement:

- the quality of goods procured is the same whether they are sold or donated;
- altruistic individuals will continue to donate in the same proportion once a market is introduced;
- when markets are banned, the price of the good is set at zero and no additional costs are required to procure the donated good;

- when markets are banned, no specific action can be done to increase supply (Moatti, p.193).

Market ban defenders are saying that if the ban is lifted the quality of organs will go down, altruistic donations will plummet and pre-existing hefty expenditures on procurement and exhortation will be wasted. Even if all of this is true, it does not mean that a market will produce fewer organs than the current system. And, as just discussed, the old Titmuss argument of diminished quality appears to no longer be operative due to technological advances.

The two vertical lines in the graph below indicates that a fixed supply of organs is available from exhortation (the 2000 kidneys vertical line for $S_{donation}$), which is less than the number of organs available were it mandatory for everyone to supply an organ (the 3000 kidneys vertical line for $S_{mandatory}$). If money is introduced as part of a market-based system (the increasing diagonal lines S_{market} or $S_{market*}$), the supply of organs will go up as more money is offered, but the demand for organs will go down as they may no longer be affordable by many people. The big question is whether a market-based system will result in the same number of people being satisfied with organ transplants as in the current exhortation-based system (the increasing diagonal line at 2000 kidneys, $S_{donation}$). Proponents of markets argue that more people will be satisfied at a lower cost per organ, i.e., the curve will look like S_{market}. Opponents argue that fewer people will be satisfied at a higher cost per organ, i.e., the curve will look like S_{market}. In addition, opponents of organ markets argue that because of the public's general revulsion at selling organs, even the 2000 kidneys currently achievable via exhortation, shown as the vertical line $S_{donation}$, will shift sharply to the left as the public eschews altruistic donation due to its confusion in their minds with the parallel (repulsive) organ market. Consequently, any introduction of an organ market will result in higher per-organ procurement costs and fewer organs – two big negatives.

These arguments are embraced by organ procurement organizations that have little reason to change the status quo. An organ market would likely shift power away from them since buyers and sellers could reach deals on the internet, register at a hospital, and conclude their transplantation business. Organ procurement organizations are bureaucracies that inherently strive to survive. Indeed, the only market-type mechanisms they are considering at all are ones that make procurement organizations the only purchasers of organs, at a monopolist set minimal price (Coleman, p.16). Such solutions would seem to actually be the worst of all worlds. People desperate enough to sell their organs would be entitled to, but the bulk of the benefit from such a sale would not accrue to them. Indeed, the economic incentive schemes considered by procurement organizations are generally geared at cadaveric donations only, with minimal proceeds paid only to the family of the donor after successful organ removal. Such markets are unlikely to thrive.

For example, until such time as the public expresses comfort with organ sales, by the creation of an organ surplus in some locale that authorizes a market, the organ procurement organizations will use the threat of diminished organ supplies to keep the market genie in its bottle. So long as opinion studies reflect values such as 93 percent objection of the French public to organ sales (Moatti, p.197), organ procurement organizations will be able to defeat organ market legislation. With this repulsion-based argument in mind, almost all bioethicists oppose an organ market. As will be seen below, though, they use proxy arguments instead of basing their opposition on repulsion.

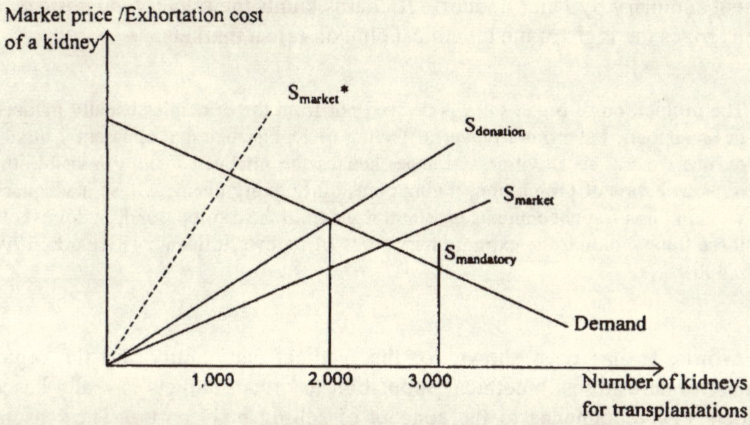

Figure I-1 Market for Organs: The Alternative View
(Moatti, p.194).

Bioethical Reasons Such as Autonomy for Banning Organ Sales

Leading bioethicists are almost unanimously opposed to the concept of permitting people to sell "spare" organs or organ parts (Caplan, "If," p.151). There is less bioethical opposition to sales of organs after death, such as by entering into a "future's contract" for one's heart or by decision of one's next of kin (Council on Ethical and Judicial Affairs, p.581). The bedrock of bioethical opposition to selling organs is that such decisions would be effectively coerced out of a need for money. A cardinal principle of bioethics is that all decisions regarding medical procedures should be based on "informed consent." Achieving this standard requires a decision that is *voluntarily* made by a *competent* person who is *fully informed* of the consequences of the decision (Shannon, p.30).

Leading bioethicist Arthur Caplan summarizes opposition to an organ market thusly:

> Creating a market in organs would give incentives to the poor and disadvantaged to sell their body parts in ways that might adversely affect their health and well being. And even if markets were restricted to sales from the dead, the potential for conflict of interest among physician and patient, family members and the

> dying would appear to threaten the ability of individuals to do with their bodies as they wish (Caplan, "If," p.151).

Astute commentators rail against the patent inconsistencies in the bioethicists' dogma, but to no avail (Richards, 1996). For example, in Caplan's second sentence quoted above he opposes markets because they "threaten the ability of individuals to do with their bodies as they wish," while in his first sentence he seeks to prevent the "disadvantaged" from doing with their bodies as they wish. An eloquent summary by Janet Radcliffe Richards taunts the *reductio ad absurdum* that characterizes the logic of the bioethical elite on organ markets:

> The prohibition of organ sales is derived not from the principles usually invoked in its support, but from a powerful feeling of repugnance that apparently numbs ordinary moral sensitivities and anaesthetizes the intellect, making invisible the obvious harms of prohibition, giving plausibility to arguments whose inadequacy would in less fraught contexts proclaim itself from the rooftops, and, in doing both these things, hiding the extraordinary force of its own influence (Richards, 1996 p.406).

In other words, as has been shown for the medical community and the organ procurement organizations, bioethical opposition to organ markets is really based on a hidden, raw repugnance to the concept of selling body parts. The reasons given (Supply Side Economics, Autonomy or Informed Consent) are merely verbal shields and linguistic costumes for gut-level opposition. To further clarify the paucity of logically defensible bioethical argument against organ markets, consider the point-counterpoint table below:

Table I-3 Bioethical Reasons Against/For Organ Sales

Bioethical Reason Against Organ Sales	Bioethical Reason For Organ Sales
Autonomy:	
Wealth disparity undermines poor's autonomy (Exploitation of the poor by the rich) Poor are too uneducated to give valid consent (Nefarious middlemen will take advantage of poor) Poor's education level too low for counseling (Poor can not be informed of the risks)	Removing sales option further reduces autonomy (Removing right to sell makes poor even worse off) Valid consent can be achieved through counseling (The trade can be regulated to ensure valid consent) Low education does not disqualify altruistic organs (Not all poor are uneducated or uninformable)
Nonmalfeasance:	
Paternalistic non-malfeasance obligation to poor (Must protect the poor from undue risks) (Transplant surgery is very dangerous)	Nonmalfeasance does not forbid altruistic donations (Poor not protected from giving organ to relative) (Poor are allowed to taker greater labor safety risks)
Beneficience:	
There is no real benefit for the poor (They will squander the money)	If poor chooses to sell, the choice must be beneficient (Not all or even most of the poor would squander)
***Justice*:**	
Unjust for organs to flow from poor to rich (Only the rich will benefit)	Justice is served by payment for organs to poor (The rich always benefit from better medical care)
Slippery Slope:	
Slippery slope to slavery and suicide for hearts (First blood sales, then kidneys, then hearts) Organ commodification demeans human dignity (Treating body parts like products is disgusting)	Regulations can prevent the slippery slope (Renewable/redundant versus vital is a hard line) Commodities have no say in destiny; not applicable (Poverty demeans dignity; getting money is uplifting)

(Richards, p.406).

As Dr. Richards opined, the bioethical objections to organ sales do not enjoy logical force. They are simply justifications for a preset abhorrence. Since the medical profession's, organ procurement organization's and bioethicist's reasons for prohibiting an organ sales market all devolve to repugnance, it is now appropriate to see what underlies this third and ultimate basis of objection.

Public Revulsion Reason for Banning Organ Sales

The American Medical Association considered revulsion at organ sales to be a consequence of the fact that "the body is part of the integrity of the person . . . [and this creates] a unique relationship between the individual and his or her own body" [so that] society prohibits individuals from selling their bodies in other contexts, such as prostitution and slavery" (Council on Ethical and Judicial Affairs, p.586). This justification, however, does not appear useful since many people sell their bodies in legal ways (models, athletes, soldiers, maids, lawyers). The point is to understand *why* society permits some ways of selling your body, and prohibits others. Dr. Richards, on the other hand, believes public revulsion at organ sales is a uniquely Western "guilt-trip," and our refusal to recognize its irrationality is a result of our strong desire not to be reminded of how unfair life can be.

> Prohibition may make things worse for the Turkish father and other desperate people who advertise their kidneys, as well as for the sick who will die for lack of them; but at least these people will despair and die quietly, in ways less offensive to the affluent and healthy, and the poor will not force their misery on our attention by engaging in the strikingly repulsive business of selling parts of themselves to repair the deficiencies of the rich (Richards 1996, p.406).

She notes that society has overcome its initial repugnance at "interracial marriage, unfeminine women and homosexuality," implying that organ sales repugnance can also be deposited in history if we squarely recognize it as an irrational prejudice and not something required by economics or bioethics. Indeed, society's repugnance might melt away if it would only come to recognize the fundamental anthropological insights of Marcel Mauss on the subject of gifts:

> The unreciprocated gift still makes the person who has accepted it inferior, particularly when it has been accepted with no thought of returning it (Mauss, p.65).

Mauss made clear, as far back as the 1920s, that there are no such things as "unilateral gifts," except to establish dominance, for the true nature of a gift is as part of an exchange "to create mutual interests, giving mutual satisfaction" (Mauss, p.82). In a similar vein, Orwell has observed that "Generosity is as painful as meanness, gratitude as hateful as ingratitude" (Orwell, p.233). In other words, repugnance may be a function of seeing the exchange of money for organs as exploitation; in fact it could be viewed much more pleasantly as an exchange of gifts.

It is impossible to predict whether society will ever overcome its repugnance at organ sales, although very limited government reimbursement of living unrelated donor expenses is beginning to achieve legal recognition in the U.S. via the "Organ Donation Improvement Act of 2001" ("Huge," p.2). Some of Dr. Richards' examples would imply that such a cultural attitude shift may be decades away at minimum. One hundred years after the end of slavery in the United States, interracial marriage was still illegal in half the American states and many Americans *still* believe it should be illegal. Forty years after the birth of the "gay rights movement," less than five countries in the world permit a gay couple to adopt a child or marry. In most of the world homosexuality is publicly deemed "repugnant," even while the Western psychological establishment considers it normal. Clearly, public attitudes on repugnance take a long time to change.

Consequently, even though an organ sales market among living donors could eliminate all shortages of lungs, livers, kidneys and pancrei, such a market is not likely to surface until public repugnance on the subject abates. Based on similar subjects, that time frame is measured in decades *after the commencement* of social agitation. Patients in need of transplants rarely have the energy to agitate. Furthermore, it will be recalled that an organ market could not satisfy society's need for hearts in any event.

Conclusion

Organ transplantation is the most effective way to extend one's life when faced with organ failure. The latest statistics show that half of all heart transplant patients worldwide, survive nearly ten years (Hosenpud et al. 2000, p.909). The longevity extends to 12 years for those who make it at least one year (Hosenpud et al. 2000, p.915). The problem is that there are not enough of the life-saving organs to meet the demand. While it is reported that about 100,000 patients need organs in the U.S. and Europe, there is a latent (unreported) demand that is approximately ten times as great.

As with other sectors in which human production falls short of social demands, a cry goes out for mechanization and technology. Perhaps mass produced bio-machines can supply the hundreds of thousands of organs needed to keep our bodies from breaking down and dying. Perhaps artificial organs can make up for the shortcomings of cadaveric donors, improved procurement infrastructure and unwelcome body parts market. But, we will never know the answers to these questions until we shed our societal repugnance and look toward "untraditional" methods of organ procurement.

Chapter II

Brave New Organs: The Status of Technological Solutions to the Problem

Chapter I demonstrated that better methods of organizing the swapping of organs among persons living and dead are unlikely to satisfy the huge million-organ-a-year needs of patients (for the US, Europe and Japan alone). Human ingenuity was especially likely to turn to technology to address this gap because organ transplantation was, itself, a creature of technology. Indeed, there is a prolific array of potential technological fixes to the organ gap. While it is impossible to definitively pick the ultimate "winning technology," it is highly likely that animal organs will be part of the transplant surgeon's armamentarium for the dying patient of the 21st century.

Introduction

There are three main kinds of technology solutions to the organ shortage problem. The first approach involves pure machines, such as the famous Jarvik-7 wholly artificial heart. The second track involves hybrid bio-artificial organs. With these a collection of specialized tissue created from DNA-driven cell duplication is used to replace a native organ, with some kind of post-transplant mechanical support. The third track involves wholly biological replacement organs, grown either in a lab from a human cell line ("organogenesis") or in an animal's body from chimeric animal-human DNA ("xenografts").

This robust array of technology development for organ replacement is itself a testament to a consensus that cadaveric donors, improved procurement infrastructure and financial incentives are inadequate solutions. In this chapter each of the different technologies will be analyzed as to which, if any of them, could satisfy society's extant and latent demand for organs.

Some Assembly Required: Status of Wholly Artificial Organs

Human efforts to replace limb body parts with artificial substitutes date to antiquity. For most of this time, artificial body parts consisted of tree branches whittled to replace a lost leg or arm. The resultant pain and discomfort from poor fitting artificial limbs is difficult to imagine. From the 16th century (for the benefit of soldiers) and especially in the 20th century – mostly in the wake of the two World Wars – increasingly sophisticated sets of hinges, springs, joints and attachments were used to establish limb functionality. With the birth of electronics and composite materials, the science of prosthetics has come closer than ever to providing analogs of the human limb. Approximately 13 million prosthetic procedures are performed in the United States annually (Presnall, p.9).

Even great boosters of electro-mechanical prosthetics don't claim to be near to a facsimile of the natural arm or leg. And it is much the same with vital organs. While artificial substitutes can replicate much of the functioning of some vital organs, they are nothing like a facsimile due to limitations that keep them external to the body. And nothing short of an internal artificial organ that works as good as the original is likely to satisfy human demand for organ transplants. (Indeed, doctors recently performed a number of hand transplants, which, if successful in the long-term, could render the prosthetic obsolete (Jones et al., p.1)).

Table II-1 History and State-of-the-Art in Wholly Artificial Body Parts

Body Part	First Used	Implant?	1999 Total	Typical Device Name
Limbs	1500	No	Millions	Jointed Limb
Limbs	1981	Yes	Thousands	Myo-electric arm
Ear	1972	Yes	7000	Cochlear Ear Implant
Eye	1960s	Yes	1M/Year	Lens Implants
Skin	1985	Yes	1000/Year	Dermagraft
Heart Valve	1960	Yes	2000K/Yr	Starr-Edwards Valve
Pacemaker	1957	Yes	100K/Yr	Cordiss
Arteries[a]	1953	Yes	10K/Yr	
Heart-Lung	1949[d]	No	2000	
Heart	1982[d]	Yes/No[b]	2000	Jarvik/Novacor
Lung	1950	No	Thousands	Iron Lungs; ECMO[e]
Kidney	1960[c]	No	50,000	Hemodialysis
Pancreas	1920s	No	Millions	Insulin Injections

[a] Body has 100,000 km of arteries, veins and capillaries.
[b] Power system is not implantable.
[c] Chronic use; acute use dates to 1943.
[d] Intended for, or de facto, temporary use as bridge to transplant.
[e] ECMO = Extra Corporeal Membrane Oxygenator.

The first artificial organ made was a kidney machine used successfully in 1944 to cleanse blood by passing it through a membrane (Porter, p.620). However, it was not until 1960 that dialysis was conceptualized as a *chronic* treatment because up to that point, surgery was needed each time a patient was hooked up. It was the relatively simple invention that year by Dr. Belding Scribner at the University of Washington of an implantable set of tubes in the forearm that permitted dialysis machines to be easily attached and detached for thrice weekly, life-long use. Some half-million patients worldwide use this method today to survive with chronic dialysis (Presnall, p.37).

By the 1950s, "iron lungs" and "heart-lung" machines were in use, again as a temporary bridge to a longer-term solution. These intrepid machines stood somewhat on the shoulders of a 1928 laboratory "heart pump" developed in England by Dale and Shuster, and a 1932 prototype "whole body perfusion device" promoted by Alexis Carrel and aviation pioneer Charles Lindbergh. A wholly artificial liver has never been made.

Despite over a half-century of practice, not a single artificial organ has been manufactured that is small and reliable enough to fit inside the body. The large number of kidney dialysis patients on the kidney transplant waiting list is evidence that patients are unwilling to live with external artificial organs if (implantable) transplants are available. Carrying or rolling around an external vital organ results in a much diminished quality of life. Among transplant professionals, the goal is for a new organ to be "forgettable."

The 'Wholly' Grail: A Total (Not Partial) Artificial Heart

There are several reasons why artificial organ technology has been most focused, albeit without success, on a total artificial heart. First, more people in the West die of heart failure than of any other disease. Second, there was a longstanding misconception of the heart as simply a mechanical pump – something that could readily be replicated by "space age technology." Third, the heart has a lyric role in human culture that tends to attract the lion's share of professional, medical and popular media attention. Finally, and in no small part due to the preceding three factors, at the insistence of the U.S. Congress, the National Institutes of Health began in the early 1960s to allocate millions of dollars a year in grants specifically for artificial heart technology (Fox and Swazey, *Spare Parts*, pp.101, 146-47). Highly effective partial cardiac assistance devices have never garnered the attention showered on largely ineffective totally artificial hearts.

The history of artificial hearts is punctuated with the names of the patients (Barney Clark, 1982; William Shroeder, 1984) and surgeons (Dr. Denton Cooley's temporary artificial heart in 1969 and Dr. William DeVries' "permanent" Jarvik-7 device in the 1980s) who pioneered the technology. Practical efforts actually began with a heart-pump project at Ohio's Cleveland Clinic initiated by a Dutch émigré, Dr. Willem Kolff, who had earlier paved the way for kidney dialysis machines with experimental models he built and tested secretly under Nazi occupation during World War II. Power was Kolff's nemesis in his efforts to develop a fully implantable heart – and it remains the primary reason there are no wholly implantable artificial hearts today, nearly half a century later. Implantable power sources are too weak to pump the heart's load of five liters a minute of blood – five times the rate of a truck's fuel pump. Compressed air appeared for years to be the best solution, even though that means the patient is stuck with an external air compressor linked to the artificial heart by tubing. More recently, electrical power supplies are becoming a feasible alternative, and a few battery-powered wine cork-sized cardiac-assistance pumps have been implanted with only a thin wire protruding through the skin (*Transplant News*, April 2000, p.7).

By 1965, the extraordinarily creative Dr. Kolff demonstrated an air compressor-powered artificial heart in a calf (about the same time, he invented a home-use Maytag washing machine and cellophane-based dialysis system to save the lives of thousands who couldn't afford hospital-based dialysis). After over a decade of animal trials, the year of the Moon Walk, 1969, also saw Dr. Denton Cooley's historic first-ever implantation of an artificial heart, albeit merely as a bridge to cadaveric heart transplantation. This artificial heart was still not entirely internal, since it was connected to a huge air compressor the size of a refrigerator. Furthermore, Cooley's and other surgeons' subsequent patients died within days or weeks of their operations, leading quickly to a moratorium on the procedures. Interestingly, the patients rarely died due to failure of the artificial heart itself, although it was often considered a contributing factor to the patients' health problems. The machines were usually ceremonially turned off by the doctors and patient families after a neurologist declared the patient brain-dead (Fox and Swazey, *Spare Parts*).

The moratorium ended with the FDA's 1981 approval of the Jarvik-7 artificial heart. This device was thought to be the pinnacle of implanted artificial heart engineering, although it still required a rolling cart of 350 pounds worth of air compressor equipment for power (eventually downsized to a backpack-sized power system). It was invented at the University of Utah by Dr. Robert Jarvik, under the tutelage of Dr. Kolff, and was eventually developed by a company called "Symbion" that Kolff and Jarvik formed. A University of Utah transplant surgeon, Dr. William DeVries, pioneered the use of the Jarvik-7 heart, and, for many years, was the only person authorized by the FDA to implant it.

A total artificial heart, such as the Jarvik-7, differs from partial cardiac assistance devices, such as pacemakers or left ventricular assistance devices ("LVADs"), in that it replaces the heart's entire pumping apparatus (left and right ventricles are surgically removed, although the atria and pulmonary valves are retained), whereas LVADs replace only the more critical left ventricular heart tissue. Until 2000, the Jarvik-7 was the only total artificial heart ever approved for permanent use. It was used as an intended permanent heart replacement just five times in the 1980s (once in Utah, three times in Kentucky and once in Sweden), with the longest surviving patient lasting nearly two years, but most of the patients succumbing after just a few months to strokes, hemorrhages and infections. It and dozens of competitive total artificial hearts have been in use ever since, but only as temporary bridges to cadaveric heart transplantation (to keep a patient on the verge of deadly heart failure alive long enough to receive a transplant). During 2000-2001, clinical trials began with miniaturized artificial hearts intended for permanent use (*Transplant News*, August 12, 2000, p.6). However, completely artificial heart technology must now compete with a growing array of competitive alternatives for failure of one or another heart function. It is not obvious that an entire new heart is needed if failing parts of the heart can be replaced instead. These competitive alternatives are explored next.

Cardiac Assistance Devices – Part of an Organ Covers Part of the Gap

The absence of any near-term prospect for wholly implantable artificial kidneys, lungs, hearts or livers – stands in sharp contrast to remarkable success in implantable cardiac *assistance* devices. Hundreds of thousands of artificial heart valves (first used in 1960), tens of thousands of cardiac pacemakers (first used in 1957) and thousands of implanted defibrillators (first used in 1980) have effectively given dead or dying hearts new life. These devices replicate specific failing functions of the heart – valve control or electrical – rather than its entire mechanical function. This makes them equivalent to an artificial heart for many patients. For example, only 2 percent of cardiac patients given an implantable defibrillator die within a year, compared to 30 percent of cardiac patients treated conventionally (Rothfeder, p.175).

Other machines, known as Left Ventricular Assist Devices, or LVADs, actually help the heart pump blood and are fully implantable except for their power supply and a pressure balancing tube. LVADs are used routinely in place of a wholly artificial heart because most of the heart's work is done by the left ventricle, and most cardiac patients suffer from left-heart failure. The left ventricle can even take over the right ventricle's job of supplying blood to the lungs in most patients with right-heart failure. However, a weakness of the LVAD is that its asymmetry necessitates a pressure-balancing tube to be run outside of the body (in addition to the power line), giving rise to risk of life-threatening infection and patient inconvenience. A wholly artificial heart balances left-side pumping with right-side pumping, as does the natural heart, thereby avoiding the pressure asymmetry problem. Consequently, a wholly artificial heart remains the holy grail.

At first blush, the progress in artificial cardiac assist devices provides hope that artificial organ technology can preempt the need for biological transplant solutions. However, on further consideration, it must be realized that 3000 people per million in Europe and America are dying of heart disease *despite* 40 years of pacemakers and 10 years of implantable defibrillators. Although lack of access to appropriate medical care and technology is a big part of the problem, also relevant is that *one third* of heart failure is not due to arrhythmias treatable with implantable devices (Rothfeder, p.7). Consequently, even if everyone who could benefit from a pacemaker or defibrillator had one, there would still be 1000 people per million dying each year of heart disease. Robert Jarvik, who now makes an implantable and transdermally-rechargeable cardiac assistance device called the "Jarvik-2000," estimates a market of only several tens of thousands of such devices (Ditlea, p.32). One of his most successful patients, Peter Houghton of England, has risen from near-death to being able to complete an 81 mile walk with the device.

Summary of Wholly Artificial Organ Technology

Wholly artificial organs do not appear likely to solve the organ shortage any time soon. This is because there are no wholly artificial organs for the liver, and no wholly implantable ones for the rest of the body. Implantable organ-*assist* devices exist only for the heart, and even these do not preclude the need for an artificial heart. While much progress is being made on implantable artificial hearts, nagging power supply problems create an opportunity for biological alternatives. Overall, wholly artificial organs for replacing failed lungs, hearts, kidneys, and livers present enough shortcomings that large numbers of transplant scientists are working to substitute dying organs for biological machines – either hybrid mechanico-biological organs, or designer organs grown to order in laboratory vats or "animal pharms."

Human-Cyborg Relations: Status of Bio-Artificial Organs

Bio-artificial organ technology arose as a solution to the dilemma of how to transplant biological organs, tissues or cells from animals into people without giving rise to rejection based on the natural immune response. The solution to this dilemma was identified as early as 1957 by Thomas Ming Swi Chang of Canada: encapsulate the foreign biology in a semi-permeable artificial membrane that prevents ingress by attacking cells of the immune system while permitting egress by the desired proteins produced by the transplant (Chang, p.249). This general concept is known as "immuno-isolation."

At present, bio-artificial organ technology does not present a realistic long-term method of dealing with the shortage of any organ except the pancreas. The current focus of bio-artificial organ technology is as a bridge to transplantation for the liver, and as a permanent, implanted pancreas. There is also interest in bio-artificial encapsulation technology to deliver transplanted brain tissues, thyroid glands and other specialized cells.

Bio-Artificial Livers

In the bridge to transplantation mode for the liver, a bedside machine houses either a whole pig liver or a package of roughly one billion porcine hepatocytes completely surrounded by an ultra-high-tech polymer membrane (Abouna 2001, p.121). This artificial liver machine is perfused with the patient's blood. As the blood passes the pig liver or pig liver cells under pressure, the detoxifying and biosynthesis functions of the liver are performed. Remarkably, whole pig livers support the body for enough time for many human livers to regenerate, and two viral hepatitis patients on the verge of death when treated with an early version of this system in 1972, were reported living 28 years later with their own, regenerated liver (Abouna 2001, p.121). The polymer membrane is specially engineered to prevent ingress by immune cells that would destroy the artificial liver. In clinical studies with humans, patients have been kept alive long enough on the bio-artificial liver (days to weeks) to receive a cadaveric liver transplant, and thereby return to normal life (Chen et al., p.358).

The bio-artificial liver also has value because of the unique ability of the liver to regenerate itself, if not cirrhotic, and if given enough time (Abouna 2001, p.120). Unfortunately, in "fulminant liver failure" the liver stops working abruptly and the person dies within days, which is too short a time for the liver to regenerate. Much of the demand for transplanted livers could be addressed by using bio-artificial livers to take the detoxification and biosynthesis load off an ailing liver long enough for it to regenerate (Abouna 2001, p.124). There would still be a significant demand for liver transplants because of patient livers that are too diseased for regeneration, due to scarring or cancer.

Growing Your Own: Status of Wholly Bio-Engineered Organs

Frustrated with technology's current inability to replicate, on a long-term, "forgettable" basis, the vital functions of the body, industry is focusing most of its artificial organ efforts on merging naturally-directed organ development with human ingenuity. These efforts take two forms: "organogenesis" and "xenografting." With organogenesis, a new organ is literally grown in a vat or structural matrix of nutrient solutions, relying on mitosis and starting with one or more cells of the desired organ. Xenografting, on the other hand, aims to modify animal organs or tissues so that rejection will not occur.

Organogenesis

Bio-engineered organs could start with the intended recipient's own cells, or with custom-designed universal human immunotolerant cells (which have been hypothesized, but never created). It is then necessary to instruct the cells to replicate and grow into the desired organ. This feat has only been accomplished to date with bones, skin and small segments of blood vessels, starting in each case with a differentiated cell of the intended new tissue type. Compared to these homogenous tissues, vital organs generally consist of many different kinds of cells. No one has figured out how to get all of the different cells of a complex existing organ to duplicate and merge into a new organ *ex vivo* or *in vivo*. However, such a feat is deemed to be feasible if assisted by a biodegradable matrix that provides three dimensional structure and sustenance to the growing organ while gradually dissolving into it (Langer and Vacanti, p.132).

The big biotechnology story of the 1990s was that it is possible to reset the clock on a differentiated cell, so that it becomes a progenitor cell once again, and can thereby spawn an entire "cloned" organism (Harris, *Clones*, p.9). However, if this "Dolly" trick were done with human cells, it would mean producing, at some point in the process, a human embryo (Harris, *Clones*, pp.46-49). There currently appears to be little prospect that public policy will permit human embryos to be created for the purpose of culling functioning organs notwithstanding the lack of moral credentials possessed by such cell masses (Harris, *Clones*, p.65). This conclusion is based on the fact that all major countries forbid laboratory manipulation of embryos older than 2-4 weeks. However, at that cut-off point, the embryos do not have developed organs that could be culled for transplantation.

By the time fetuses have cullable organs – 24 weeks to 32 weeks depending on the organ – it is, at present, difficult to obtain societal permission to sacrifice them for organs. Interestingly, there is an ethical consensus that a fetus may be sacrificed to save the mother's life. An unexplored issue is whether this consensus will hold when the sacrifice is planned for reasons of organ harvesting to save the life of the male or female cell donor, rather than an accidental consequence of a pregnancy with no ulterior self-serving justification.

It may be possible to beat the fetus-organ dilemma by harvesting organ "buds" during the first trimester of fetal development. Such fetuses might be either auto-generated clones, or come from third party abortions. Such "buds" are very small (few millimeters) beginnings of organs, and currently lack viability outside the fetal environment. However, it is possible that they could be nested in *ex vivo* matrix structures and grown to the point of transplantability. As of 2001, this possibility is still too futuristic to engender serious ethical debate.

The tissue engineering challenge is to overcome all ethical objections to human embryo/fetus manipulation by learning how to instruct a progenitor cell to differentiate into *only* the desired organ. In this way, it can legitimately be claimed that an embryo/fetus is not being created, just a spare organ. Somewhat equivalently, there are searches underway for organ-specific progenitor cells that, if properly nurtured, would grow into an entire organ (Reubinoff et al., p.399). Such cells are thought to exist because cells formed immediately after fertilization are "totipotent," meaning they can differentiate into every kind of cell in the body and carry the DNA instructions on how to do so.

As an initial zygote divides into the blastocyst stage and beyond, rudimentary cell differentiation begins to occur. Some cells begin to appear and function differently than other cells. This process of differentiation begins around the 3rd week and continues until a small mass of cells begins beating (the heart) in the 4th week, engaging in biosynthesis (the liver) in the 5th week, and so on. Consequently, there must be biochemical instructions in totipotent cells that "turn on" particular subsets of DNA associated with the specific functionality of a vital organ (Reubinoff et al., p.399). Once those subsets are triggered, and a differentiated "vital organ" cell is produced, it replicates itself until there is enough of a critical mass of such cells to constitute an "organ," commencing in the 6th week with a "proto-organ" or "bud." However, the initial process of a progenitor cell triggering a subset of DNA must also be repeated one or more times since vital organs consist of more than one type of differentiated cells. Lungs, for example, contain at least forty different cell types in an exquisitely interlaced structure of air sacs, blood vessels, mesenchyme, and millions of bronchial branches (A. Fishman 1998, pp.91-95). Thus, either some of the initially differentiated cells themselves sub-differentiate, and/or some of the original progenitor cells that differentiated into one type of vital organ cell, also differentiate into other types of cells found in a given vital organ.

The answers to these fundamentally important questions to organogenesis are, as of 2002, almost entirely unknown. Scientists do not know what causes an original progenitor stem cell to differentiate. Scientists do not know why such cells differentiate into cells of one or another type of organ. And scientists do not know whether the various cells of a vital organ are created from a single organ progenitor cell or from multiple differentiations of a totipotent stem cell. Clearly, even the basic theory of organogenesis is at a rudimentary phase.

All such progenitor cell efforts, also known as "stem cell" efforts, are in their infancy. No organ-specific progenitor or stem cells have yet been found, and no one has ever instructed a whole-body stem cell (such as one of the first cells formed after an egg is fertilized or a cell is cloned) to differentiate into a specific vital organ. Consequently, only by virtue of lucky breakthroughs will organogenesis make any near-term difference in the organ gap. One such breakthrough would be if an already differentiated cell of a specific organ, such as the heart, could be extracted via biopsy (or cultured into various immunotolerant strains) and chemically reprogrammed to regenerate its entire organ in an appropriate structural matrix. Similarly, as mentioned above, a breakthrough could involve extracting an organ "bud" from a first trimester fetus and getting it to grow into a mature organ in a structural matrix. These breakthroughs would avoid many of the unknowns about how to trigger totipotent cells to differentiate. On the other hand, it may well turn out to be easier to differentiate a totipotent cell and to get it to grow into a transplantable organ outside the body in a structural matrix. Absent such scientific leaps, organogenesis lies well in the future.

Xenotransplantation

Compared with organogenesis, xenotransplantation, the transplantation of organs or tissues from one species to another, is far advanced. Dozens of humans have participated in successful xenotransplantation clinical trials for pancreatic (Groth and Breimer, p.812) and liver failure (Abouna 1997, p.785; Lysaght and Aebischer, p.76), and hearts have been transplanted from pigs to primates without unmanageable rejection. However, all of the human trials involve temporary treatments, as a bridge until the native organ recovers or an allograft becomes available. There has yet to be a long-term transplant of an animal organ into a person or from one species into another.

The key to a successful xenograft is to safely prevent the immune system of the recipient from destroying the graft. At the cellular level, each species' immune system recognizes certain proteins on the surface of another species' organ as being drastically "not-self." The more divergent the species are in the evolutionary tree, the more "not-self" the graft's proteins will appear and the more aggressive will be the immune system's attack. Put simply, cross-species rejection is a huge amplification of our body's natural and desired antibody reaction to foreign bacteria and viruses.

The way to minimize cross-species rejection is to create animals with "humanized" or "de-animalized" proteins on the surface of their transplantable organs. This is accomplished by using genetic engineering on an animal zygote to alter or "knock-out" the genes that code in DNA for the surface proteins triggering rejection (Vanhove et al., p.30). Once animals have been produced that lack the undesired proteins, they are mated or cloned until a homogeneous herd for the genetically engineered trait is created ("Transgenic," p.365). This combination of animal husbandry with genetic technology has been proven feasible with pig hearts transplanted into baboons (Platt and Lin, p.7), and is now immediately ready for human trials.

The biochemical differences among species are multitudinous, and the interactions among these molecular biological systems are, at least at present, complex beyond the realm of human comprehension. The gross differences observed between species at the level of the observable characteristics are mirrored in countless differences at the level of amino acid combinations. Even differences observable by a child – such as the consequences of a horizontal versus a vertical posture for blood flow – may be important for long-term xenotransplant survival due to hemodynamic consequences. Differences wrought by evolution across the species in terms of enzymes, hormones, antibodies, interleukins, adhesion molecules, cytokines, eicosanoids, and countless other proteins and peptides are certain to have some impact on the ability of a person to survive over time with a xenograft (Friend and Soin, p.111). Is xenotransplantation in fact ready to become a permanent player on the medical scene? To answer this question it is necessary to take a deeper look at the science and technology underlying xenotransplantation.

The Science of Xenotransplantation

Of course people knew for millennia that larger mammals (such as pigs, sheep and cattle) had vital organs that were, in most observable respects, similar to those of humans. Consequently, soon after organ suturing techniques were mastered, surgeons attempted to save patient lives with transplants of animal organs. Those pioneering xenografts failed rapidly. Table II-2 below describes the world experience with implanted whole-organ clinical xenotransplantation, listing the longest survival for each organ and donor in a given year. It is interesting to note that the number of xenotransplants falls off for each organ soon after significant new survival records are established. The reason for this is that the new survival records are associated with the introduction of a new generation of immunosuppression drugs. These new drugs make multi-year survival possible with human-to-human transplants, thereby creating little interest in doing further xenotransplants, the large majority of which provide only days of additional survival.

Table II-2 Longest Survival for Various Years, Donors and Xenografts

Year	Donor	Organ	Survival	Note
1905	Rabbit	Kidney	16 days	
1906	Pig	Kidney	<3 days	
1906	Goat	Kidney	<3 days	
1910	Monkey	Kidney	<2 days	
1923	Sheep	Kidney	<9 days	
1964	Chimp	Kidney	9 months	1st generation immunosuppressant available
1964	Baboon	Kidney	2 months	
1964	Chimp	Heart	2 hours	
1966	Chimp	Liver	<1 day	
1968	Sheep	Heart	<1 hour	
1968	Pig	Heart	4 minutes	
1969	Chimp	Heart	4 hours	
1969	Chimp	Liver	9 days	
1969	Baboon	Liver	<1 day	
1970	Baboon	Liver	3 days	
1971	Baboon	Liver	3 days	
1974	Chimp	Liver	14 days	
1977	Baboon	Heart	5 hours	
1977	Chimp	Heart	4 days	
1984	Baboon	Heart	20 days	Cyclosporine available
1992	Pig	Heart	1 day	
1992	Baboon	Liver	70 days	
1993	Baboon	Liver	26 days	
1993	Pig	Liver	<2 days	

Source: Taniguchi and Cooper, pp.778-79

By the 1990s, a science of xenotransplantation had evolved, which defined four stages of xenograft failure. Recent scientific progress relevant to each of these four stages now propels optimism that xenotransplantation will not be a "flash in the pan" like the Jarvik-7 heart, but instead a practical new way to save patient lives.

First Stage of Failure: Hyperacute Rejection ("HAR")

In this phase, certain human (and other Old World primate) cells called "xenoreactive antibodies" lock onto a sugar in xenograft organs which coats the endothelial lining of blood vessels in all lower mammals and New World monkeys (Cooper and Lanza 2000, p.71). Within minutes of when this molecule-to-molecule coupling occurs, a set of "complement" molecules collects near the site of coupling. The complement molecules somehow attract, and are followed by "natural killer" and other destructive cells, which slice into the endothelial cells lining the blood vessels of the graft. Within hours, the graft has been sliced (lysed in medical terminology) into a poorly differentiated bloody mass of cells (Cooper and Lanza 2000, p.57). Hyperacute rejection is also called "humoral" rejection because resources throughout the body are called upon to attack the xenograft. For example, the xenoreactive antibodies that attack the graft are pre-formed (they actually comprise one percent of all of our antibodies) and circulate throughout the body, usually limiting their attacks to alien microbes that enter our body via food (Squinto and Fodor, p.660).

First Stage of Xeno-Success: Transgenic Animals

While there are a number of pharmacological methods of beating back HAR, the greatest prospect for success lies with genetic modification of animal donor organs. In order to defeat HAR it is necessary to deal with the human body's strong distaste for the sugar found on the lining of animal organs (Cooper and Lanza 2000, pp.80-81). With a transgenic animal, genetic engineering is practiced upon the animal's precursor blastocyst, or that of its ancestors. The genetic engineering consists of adding a new gene or blocking the full operation of an existing gene. This is accomplished by injecting into one of the cells of a blastocyst many copies of a gene fragment spliced from the DNA of another species. Remarkably, a small percentage of the time, one or more copies of the injected gene fragment inserts itself somewhere in one of the helical DNA chromosomes, finds itself replicated billions of times in each of the full grown animal's cells, and is actually able to direct the production of a specific protein product. So long as the transgenic animal is fertile and passes on its spliced-in gene fragment, man has created a new animal breed. The science of transgenic animals is understood well enough that some goats have been engineered to not only produce badly needed complex proteins for pharmaceutical purposes, but to do so through their breast milk to facilitate the logistics and economics of collecting this "bio-drug."

HAR can be overcome by creating special breeds of pigs that have been "de-animalized" with regard to the endothelial lining of their organs. Such "transgenic" pig hearts transplanted into conventionally immunosuppressed cynomolgus monkeys survived an average of 40 days, compared to 55 minutes for non-transgenic xenografts (Cozzi et al., p.677). This study, carried out by the U.K. drug company Imutran, proves that transgenic pig technology has overcome the first hurdle to xenotransplantation. In short, the creation of the first transgenic animal does indeed face severe technological obstacles. However, we know that these can be overcome, and once they have, effective transgenesis becomes simply a matter of good animal husbandry.

Second Stage of Failure: Delayed Xenograft Rejection

Delayed xenograft rejection ("DXR"), which typically occurs 1-5 days after xenografting, results from newly produced, *graft-induced* xenoreactive antibodies wreaking some of the same kind of havoc described in Stage One, above (Cooper and Lanza 2000, p.68). DXR is not as severe as the HAR Stage because the HAR Stage involved *pre-formed* xenoreactive antibodies. With pre-formed antibodies, it takes literally seconds or minutes for damage to be inflicted, and there are many more of these antibodies present (Cooper and Lanza 2000, p.63).

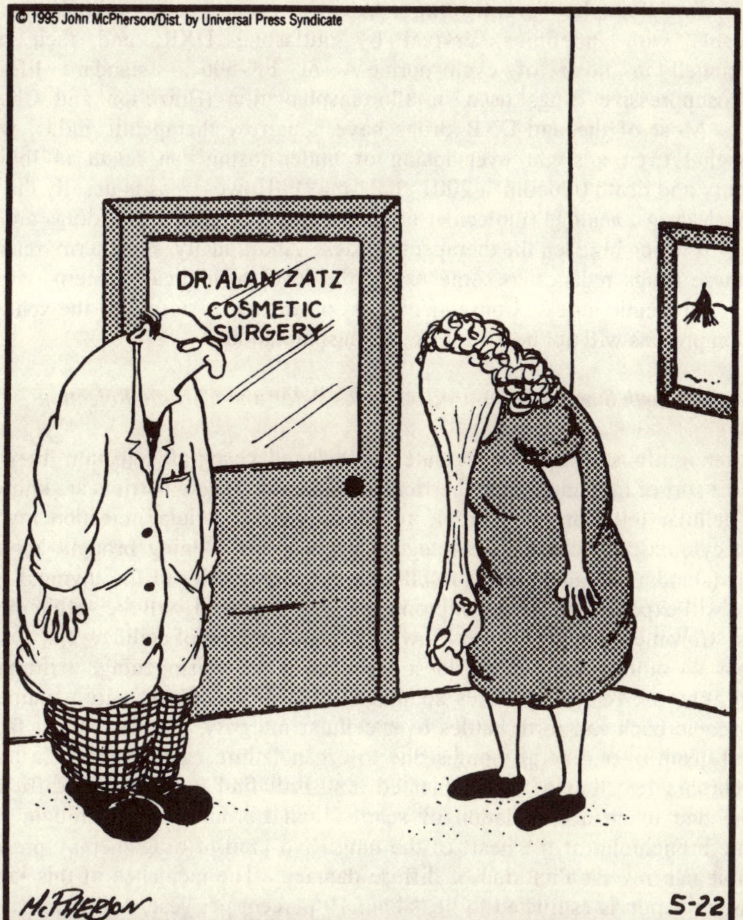

"Unfortunately, Carolyn, your body has rejected your face lift."

Second Stage of Success: Anti-Pyrimidine Biosynthesis Drugs

Researchers have enjoyed considerable success in getting xenografts past DXR (Brazelton and Cheung, p.504). Short-term therapy with immunosuppressive drugs different from those used in allotransplantation appears to break the back of DXR within about 30 days, thus providing an opportunity for some immune system accommodation to the xenograft and for a settling down of the inflamed endothelium.

A number of drugs were developed in the late 1980s and early 1990s that demonstrated remarkable success in getting cross-species xenografts to survive DXR. For example, several drugs provided cross-species animal-to-animal transplants with indefinite survival by outlasting DXR, and then being discontinued in favor of cyclosporine-A or FK-506 – standard life-long immunosuppressive drugs used in allotransplantation (Brazelton and Cheung, p.504). Most of the anti-DXR drugs have a narrow therapeutic index, which means that even a slight over-dosing or under-dosing can result in toxicity, morbidity and death (Goodman 2001 et al., p.49). However, as is usually the case with such drugs, analogs (molecular-modifications or versions of a drug) are then developed which broaden the therapeutic index. Additionally, short-term treatment with these drugs reduces to some extent the level of clinical concern with the narrow therapeutic index. Consequently, it appears as if Phase 2 of the xenograft rejection process will not be a bar to xenotransplantation.

Third and Fourth Stages of Failure: Acute Cellular and Chronic Rejection

Once xenografts surmount hyperacute and delayed xenograft rejection, they face the same sort of immune-system barriers as allografts. These barriers are known as acute cellular rejection and chronic rejection. Acute cellular rejection involves abrupt cytotoxic attacks on the integrity of an organ's lining brought about by T-cells (standard immune system cells generated primarily in the thymus). The patient will experience severe symptoms and, left untreated, will die within days or weeks. Chronic rejection is a very low-level, gradual kind of cellular rejection that happens so quietly the patient doesn't realize what is happening. Ultimately, though, chronic rejection causes so much scarring and fibrosis from numerous microscopic back-and-forth battles over cellular integrity, that the patient faces a gradual death over several months due to organ failure. For example, a patient with chronic rejection of a transplanted lung will find it ever more difficult to breathe due to an accumulation of scarred and fibrous tissues throughout the delicate bronchioles at the heart of the lung. No kind of drug therapy presently available can reverse this kind of diffuse damage. The incidence of this kind of chronic rejection is estimated to be "about 10 percent per year, with a prevalence by 10 years of virtually 100 percent" (Pierson and Miller, p.88).

Third and Fourth Stages of Success: Ever Better Immunosuppressives and Monitoring

Once a patient is bridged to the Third and Fourth Stages of rejection, then the same drugs that work for human-to-human transplants, will also work for animal-to-human transplants.

Table II-3 Summary Table of Four Stages of Xenograft Rejection

Number	**Name**	**Duration**	**Solution**
1	HAR	Hours	Transgenic Modification of Animal
2	DXR	Days	Anti-Pyrimidine Drugs; Malononitriloamides; Xeno-Thromboregulatory Agents
3	Acute	Weeks	Cyclosporine or FK-506
4	Chronic	Years	Better Patient Monitoring; 4th Generation Immunosuppressants

There is plenty of evidence of greater success in battling acute cellular rejection. Survival times for organ allotransplants are now routinely measured in years. This clearly shows that, for most patients, acute cellular rejection can be managed successfully.

The growth of a multi-billion dollar market for anti-rejection drugs has fueled competition among drug companies to develop ever more effective immunosuppressants. Generally speaking, each new generation of drugs improves on its predecessors in two ways: (1) fewer toxic side effects, and (2) greater specificity in suppressing only that part of the immune system that is involved in acute cellular rejection (not the entire body's immune system). These improvements will help minimize the toxic side effects of drugs such as Cyclosporine-A, which include a high incidence of diabetes and lymphoma, as well as the risk of death due to opportunistic infections gone wild in an over-immunosuppressed patient. FK-506 is a third generation immunosuppressive with a safer and more effective therapeutic profile than second generation Cyclosporine-A (which itself was a huge improvement over first generation approaches such as azathioprine and high-dose steroid regimes). Numerous fourth generation immunosuppressants are now working their way through clinical trials.

Evidence of success against chronic rejection is harder to come by. Allotransplant survival rates for hearts and lungs fell below 10-20 percent after ten years, with little change during the 1990s. Worse, there is no effective means of reversing the scarring and fibrosis caused by chronic rejection. However, during the 1990s, clinicians became ever more vigilant in closely monitoring their transplant patients via periodic organ performance tests and biopsies to nip chronic rejection in the bud with heightened immunosuppression. This kind of close vigilance, coupled with more selective immunosuppressant drugs, is expected to extend organ survival (Pierson and Miller, p.88).

New kinds of chronic problems can be envisaged with xenografts, such as those from illnesses due to interactions between cellular byproducts of animal and human organs, or decay of the xenograft due to the shorter lifespan of a pig. These new problems, however, may simply lead to new modes of chronic disease management – additional medications or improved transgenic modifications to eliminate adverse pig-human peptide interactions, and serial transplants to address failing xenografts.

In the final analysis, when a patient cures a disease with a transplant, they are in effect trading one disease for another – acute and chronic rejection. The hope is that the new disease will be easier to manage than the old disease. The burgeoning waitlists for organ transplants demonstrate that both the patients, and their doctors, believe this is in fact true. The Four Stages of Success experienced by xeno and allotransplantation shows that there is likely to be at hand a means of providing enough organ transplant cures for all who want them.

Realtechnik and Realpolitik: Why Xenografts Will Win

The previous section on the *Science of Xenotransplantation* has shown that xenografts are technically much more like allografts than they are like wholly artificial hearts. No new breakthroughs are necessary to make a xenograft work. Breeding animals transgenically to avoid hyper-acute rejection, and reliance upon short-term and long-term immunosuppressant drugs for surmounting delayed xenograft and acute cellular rejection, will, in all likelihood, provide patients during the next few years with a reasonable shot at an extended life-span. While new medical problems may well crop up over a period of months or years as a result of the interaction between myriad animal and human proteins and peptides, to date such problems are only hypothetical (Friend and Sohn, p.111). Such hypothetical problems are unlikely to stop the drive to employ xenografts, if for no reason other than as a bridge to an allotransplant. And, if such problems fail to materialize, or turn out to be readily managed with known pharmaceuticals, then xenografts will transmogrify into *de facto* permanent organ transplants.

In one respect, however, xenografts are more like wholly artificial organs than like allografts. This relates to supply. As with manufactured organs, there is no problematic *a priori* limit on the number of xenografts that can be produced. Pigs have been favored as xenograft sources not only because of their striking homology in size of organ to man, but because they have large litters and short periods of immaturity (Korsgren et al., p.116). Over 90 million pigs are slaughtered each year for food (Squinto and Fodor, p.660). It should therefore be readily possible to produce transgenic pigs and explant their organs in the quantities needed to satisfy even the latent demand for vital organs, at most 4000 pigs per million persons, or 4 million pigs a year for the North Atlantic Region.

The following table summarizes the findings of this book thus far regarding the feasibility of various alternative solutions to the organ gap:

Table II-4 Ability of Various Technologies to Satisfy Latent Organ Demand

	Heart	**Lung**	**Liver**	**Kidney**	**Pancreas**
Cadaveric Donors	Not enough	Possible if required by law	Possible if required by law	Possible if required by law	Possible if required by law
Living Donors	Impossible	Possible if required or sales allowed	Possible if required or sales allowed	Possible if required or sales allowed	Possible if required or sales allowed
Wholly Artificial Organs	Possible but not pleasant	Impossible for now	Impossible for now	Impossible for now	Possible in 5 years
Partial Artificial Organs	Possible for some of demand	Impossible for now	Impossible for now	Impossible for now	Possible now
Bio-Artificial Organs	Impossible for now	Impossible for now	Ok now as bridge	Possible in 5 years	Possible in 5 years
Organo-Genesis	Impossible for now	Impossible for now	Impossible for now	Impossible for now	Impossible for now
Xeno-Graft	Possible in 5 years	Impossible for now	Possible in 5 years	Possible in 5 years	Possible in 5 years

The foregoing table indicates that for all organs except the heart, extant and latent demand for new organs could be satisfied by new laws that mandated organ harvesting death procedures and/or giving up spare organs to those in need. This same demand is also likely to be satisfied by new laws that permit the selling of spare organs. None of these solutions will be adopted because of prevailing attitudes which resist granting governments greater control over individuals, and which are dead-set against "body part" markets. The only other solution for these organs are xenotransplants, either *en toto* or as part of a bioartificial package.

The foregoing table also indicates that in regard to hearts, there are only two alternatives capable of addressing the latent demand: wholly or partially artificial devices with an external power source, or xenografts. As a matter of *realtechnik*, there is doubt as to whether wholly or partial artificial hearts will succeed as well (meaning forgettable by the patient), as quickly, and as inexpensively as xenografts. Hence, xenotechnology companies are certain to compete to win at worst a share, and at best nearly all, of a potentially huge market.

For lungs, livers, kidneys and pancrei, there will be big doubts for years to come as to whether (1) living people will agree to donate their organs in sufficient number to help their fellow humans with end-stage organ failure; (2) governments will ever permit organ markets, and (3) governments will mandate cadaveric transplants. Thus, as with the heart market, xenotechnology companies have plenty of motivation to compete against these "phantoms" to win all or at least a share of these large markets.

It is not that xenotransplantation is the *only* solution to the extant and latent demand for vital organs. It is, that as a matter of *realpolitik* and *realtechnik*, xenotransplantation is a likely solution. At a bare minimum, xenotransplantation is certain to vie to be one of a set of solutions for escaping end-stage organ failure. And it may well be the best positioned contender for most favored solution, because of its advantages in quantity, quality (forgettability) and near-term availability.

The public itself has a large say as to the outcome of the competition between xenotransplantation and its alternatives. If government funding and insurance reimbursement of artificial hearts is liberal, then it is more likely that artificial hearts could beat xenotransplantation out of the heart market. If the government permits organ markets, or is willing to create an organ "draft," then it is likely that living and cadaveric transplants will beat xenotransplantation out of the rest of the vital organ market. But if government does nothing, then xenotransplantation will claim at least part of these markets.

Why should the public care? Xenotransplantation alone poses "externality costs" such as pandemic health risks through xenogeneic viruses (chapter III *infra*). If the public does nothing, it makes a *de facto* statement that it is unconcerned about these risks, or that there is nothing that it can do about them. But if the public is concerned, then there are things that can be done to kill xenotransplantation in its infancy. The question is, "should the public be concerned?"

Contrary to the problems faced by wholly artificial organs, there is no miniaturization or power-supply problem with implanting xenografts. They are designed by nature to be carried inside a body. Contrary to the problems faced by organogenesis technology, there is no fundamental breakthrough needed for xenografts to work. They are working already in non-human primates and as bridges to transplantation in humans. The technical challenges facing xenografts are incremental skirmishes in an ongoing battle against rejection. These are exactly the same kinds of skirmishes that allotransplant technology fought from the 1950s to the 1990s, and has largely conquered, provided patients comply with their medication regimen.

Xenografting can satisfy humanity's demand for organs because the technology is virtually available, and it can produce as many desired organs as are cultivated through specially bred animal herds (Onishi et al., p.1188). But there is a price to be paid for this abundant means of extending human life. The price is a risk of introducing new viruses into human society, viruses that "hitchhike" into our bloodstreams from animal organs and cause disease – possibly even triggering horrible pandemics. Is this a risk worth taking? Who should decide? How this interplay between public and private interests gets settled will determine if xenografting is an illusory solution to the organ shortage, or the objective of medicine in the 21st century and beyond.

Conclusion

Scientific success has spurred organ demand to today's level of severe organ shortages. It is not that more people are dying of organ failure, it is that due to success of transplantation, it has become reasonable to refer ever larger sets of end-stage organ failure patients for transplantation. This process can be expected to repeat itself – as the operation becomes ever safer it becomes a reasonable medical solution for larger sets of patients, including patients at less terminal stages of their disease process.

Today, there are sharp limits on who can avail themselves of transplantation due to the limited number of organs. But, as organ limits fade before technological advances, ever larger numbers of patients are sure to want access to an option that will postpone death and improve the quality of their lives. It is not unreasonable to expect the large majority of people to have one or more organ transplants during their lives to treat various medical conditions. After all, everyone will face one or more life-threatening diseases, and most zero in on a specific organ to cause death. This quanta of demand can be solved only with the tools of mass production – either on a factory assembly line for plastic organs or on "pharm" assembly line for xenografts.

Because animal-bred organs are significantly ahead in development of implantable artificial organs, we can reasonably expect xenografts to take center stage as the best technical solution to society's organ shortage problem. Whether the technically best solution is also the wisest solution depends on a societal calculus that spans risk assessment, medical ethics and philosophy. The first prong of this calculation involves risk assessment. What dangers are posed by xenotransplantation? What dampers may rightfully temper the excitement of transplant surgeons and terminal patients desperate for the tools to extend threatened lives?

Chapter III

Look Before You Leap: Technological Risks of Xenotransplantation

The previous two chapters demonstrated that a vast number of people could significantly prolong their lives with organ transplants, and that xenografts were the most realistic near-term solution to addressing that vital need. The radical new solution of using transgenic animal parts to solve the organ shortage brings with it some new public policy concerns. This chapter will discuss the foremost concern: the hypothetical ability of xenografts to cause new epidemics.

In chapter IV, the discussion will turn to other kinds of risks, such as the harm that xenotransplantation causes to animals and the socio-psychological consequences of chimerism. With this foundation in place, it will then be possible to address which bioethical and regulatory regime is most appropriate for xenotransplantation, given the balance of private interests and public risks at play. Notwithstanding the progress in the scientific feasibility of overcoming evolution's boundaries to organ sharing, "social acceptability may ultimately be a more significant barrier to xenotransplantation than immunology" (Evans and Manninen, p.367).

Introduction

Infectious diseases arise from microscopic organisms, or fragments of such life, which interact with cells in ways that cause dysfunction to occur. The microscopic organisms are called bacteria, if they can reproduce on their own (outside of a host cell), and are called viruses if they need to commandeer the DNA of another cell to affect reproduction. Recently, mere fragments of protein, called prions, have been found to cause disease (Prusiner, 1995). These entities reproduce purely enzymatically, without any genetic code at all. All of these different kinds of disease "vectors" can cause cells to fail in some way that results in illness or death to a larger host organism.

It is important to remember that these microbial disease vectors may act like innocent bystanders and simply not fit in with any part of a larger host, or may be promptly vanquished by the immune system of a host. Finally, some microscopic organisms are actually helpful to a host, such as bacteria in the human gastrointestinal tract that help to digest food. All life is a random game of ever-changing combinatorial biochemistry in which an incomprehensibly diverse array of big strings of molecules called proteins bump into each other. The close proximity brings molecular electro-mechanical interaction with one of four outcomes – no attraction, attraction but no second-order effects, attraction with healthy second-order effects, and attraction with unhealthy second-order effects. Healthy second-order effects have included the evolution of ever more complex plant and animal life from lifeless proteins – our DNA is in large part the aggregation of viral genetic code assimilated over countless eons as the viruses passed through cell membranes. Unhealthy second-order effects are diseases.

If harmful microbes are passed from one host to another, such as among children in a school, they are considered infectious. An epidemic is declared when the infectious disease appears to be causing a lot of illness or death compared to some historical norm for the condition. A pandemic is declared when the epidemic spans global distances. The acceptability of xenotransplantation depends critically on agreement that it will not cause a pandemic. To meet this criterion it must be shown both that (1) animal screening systems can create xenografts that are free of knowable harmful viruses, and (2) that if xenogeneic viral infections nevertheless do manifest themselves in patients, there are socially acceptable methods to prevent such infections from spreading to a broader population (Michaels 2001, p.130). Because it is not possible to know all viruses, the acceptability of xenotransplantation ultimately turns on the moral legitimacy of forms of bio-surveillance that go well beyond current practices.

Blood Sucking Host Hoppers: Zoonotic and Xenogeneic Bugs

A bacteria, virus or prion may cause disease in one species, but not another, and even in one individual or host within a species, but not another, due to the multudinous differences that exist on the level of molecular biology among living things. Even the most horrific diseases visited upon man – such as smallpox, plague and AIDS – serendipitously spare many individuals or afflict a differential course of disease upon infected "non-progressors." The disease vector must "lock onto" some three dimensional piece of a molecule in a host in order to have any biological effect at all – much as a key must fit a lock in order to open a door. However there is a virtually infinite array of variation in three dimensional molecular structures across all life forms. Even within a single species, such as *homo sapiens*, there is great random variation and mutated versions present in nearly every important molecule (Cavalli-Sforza, Menozzi and Piazza, p.19). Since the microbial "keys" must fit the host "locks" rather precisely, it is a rare event that such a fit occurs at all, and even rarer that the fit is followed by the cellular-level rampage we call disease. Most rare of all would be a microbial "key" that fits cells in every member of a species, and always produces disease. This is so rare because no two members of a species are ever precisely alike at the level of molecular biology.

Notwithstanding the long odds faced by disease vectors, there are enough of them constantly mutating their three dimensional structure that sooner or later they achieve some measure of success. The best case for the disease vector is high infectivity and minimum mortality for their host – in this way the disease vector can replicate to the highest possible number. The worst case for the disease vector is low infectivity and high mortality for host – in these cases the disease vector will not achieve much prevalence. But microbes are not sentient, and hence they simply wreak such havoc on such scales as their molecular keys randomly encode. The hepatitis B virus has clearly mastered the "high infectivity, minimum mortality" game. It has infected perhaps half of the human race, and yet, less than ten percent of those infected become chronic carriers, with a minority of those suffering serious illness (still enough to kill millions). When it does cause death, it usually does so only after decades of peaceful co-existence with its human host, enabling it to be innocently retransmitted many times without the host's awareness. This was before Dr. Blumberg's development of the hepatitis B test and vaccine. Versions of the virus exist in several animal species, yet there is no evidence that the virus leapt any species barrier, despite the fact that it can be found in insects that prey on humans. It is one of the simplest viruses in genetic structure, and yet science has no idea why its epidemiology is quite different in men and women (Blumberg, pp.178-82). Clearly, with infectious agents, we are dealing with amazingly complex "lock and key" mechanisms. In the totality of their behavior, endemic viruses such as hepatitis B appear able to outfox the collective wisdom of humanity.

For the same reasons that xenotransplantation is possible at all, namely the partial morphological and biochemical homology among animal species, it should not be surprising that occasionally disease vectors will function in more than one species. Some disease vector "keys" have more "master key" characteristics than others, and are able to open cellular "locks" across more than one species. Nevertheless, very few disease vector "keys" are able to both open cellular "locks" across a species boundary *and* wreak havoc with the new species host (Michaels 2001, p.129). This is because it requires one level of biochemical compatibility for a disease vector to simply dock with a three dimensional molecule in a host; it takes yet a further level of biochemical compatibility to know how to "short-circuit the wiring" of a cell, or to otherwise interfere with some important aspect of a host's physiology. The difficulty of achieving this double-effect is evidenced by the paucity of diseases that harm both animals and man, notwithstanding our close proximity over the millennia. Disease vectors do arise that infect multiple species but cause illness and/or death in only one species, e.g., man. If this microbe is also transmissible among hosts, an epidemic will arise. Examples include the following:

- HIV is endemic and harmless in our closest animal relative, chimpanzees.
- The influenza pandemic of 1918, which killed 20 million people, was a virus that was endemic and harmless in pigs and birds (Clark, p.139).

When a disease vector passes from an animal species to humans it is called "zoonotic," and the resulting disease is a "zoonosis." Hence, both HIV and the flu are zoonoses. Every year new variants of type A and type B influenza arise from domestic and wild fowl in China and other parts of Asia (Kaiser and Hayden, p.112). While the birds are unaffected by the viruses, close proximity with farmers results in viral transmission into humans who lack pre-formed antibodies against the annually-changing chemical structure ("Avian," p.5). Millions of people take ill each year due to this zoonosis. Public health officials go to Asia each spring to identify the zoonotic threat in advance, and to identify the new shape of the flu virus (Wall Street Journal, p.A15). Vaccine developers then work overtime all summer to have flu vaccines ready for the winter flu season. The vaccines place harmless fragments of the zoonotic virus into our bloodstream so that we will develop antibodies against it. Then, when exposed to the virus, our bodies have millions of pre-formed antibodies against it, and can vanquish the virus before it makes us ill.

A xenogeneic (a synonym is xenozoonotic) disease is a zoonosis that arises from xenotransplantation. A xenogeneic disease (also called a xenosis) would probably never occur without xenotransplantation because such viruses were either (1) unlikely to cross the transmission barrier without direct transplantation (as a hitchhiker on a xenograft) into a human, or (2) unlikely to surpass the human immune system without the immunosuppression that accompanies transplantation (Michaels 2001, p.130). Consequently, with xenotransplantation, society may be creating new zoonoses. Xenogeneic zoonoses ("xenozoonoses") are animal-to-human viruses made possible by the technology of xenotransplantation.

The first pig-to-human heart transplant has already occurred (in India). The responsible surgeon, Dhani Baruah, a fellow of the Royal College of Surgeons working at the Glasgow Royal Infirmary, believes "the concerns about pig-borne diseases infecting humans are also surmountable problems" and that "it is more unethical to withhold [pig hearts] from dying patients" (Rogers, p.7). The 32-year-old patient, Purno Saikia, was facing death and gained only one week of life from the pig heart before succumbing to a brain infection, possibly as a result of excess immunosuppression due to the powerful chemicals he was given to forestall rejection of the xenograft (Rogers, p.7). A month earlier, a 39-year-old American woman recovered walking ability less than a month after being the first stroke victim to be treated with a transplant of millions of brain cells from foetuses of Yorkshire pigs (*Transplant News*, October 31, 1999, p.10; Young, p.15). Dozens of patients at Baylor University in Texas and at Cedars Sinai in Los Angeles began in 1999 receiving a procedure called xenoperfusion in which their blood is perfused extracorporeally through a pig's liver, or cells from a pig's liver, until a liver is available for transplantation (Rowland, p.1). *Consequently, the xenogeneic disease genie – if it is a real problem – is very quickly slipping out of its bottle*, with thus far no known adverse effects. It is toward an ascertainment of just how real this problem is, and the magnitude of the attendant risks, that we now turn.

Theoretical Likelihood of Xenogeneic Diseases

The theory of *xenogeneic* disease transmission begins with the apparent ease by which *primate* viruses infect man (simian foamy virus infects man via scratches or bites to animal handlers) and with potentially devastating results (such as the AIDS pandemic generally believed to have emanated from simian HIV) (Heneine et al., p.403). Scientists with the world's largest baboon breeding facility, the Southwest Foundation for Biomedical Research, point out that baboons also harbor viruses that cause leukemia and T-cell lymphomas and that human T-cell lymphotropic virus (HTLV) "probably arose from cross-species transmission from non-human primates" (Allan, p.62).

Primate-based theoretical arguments regarding disease likelihood can be countered by claiming that only animals distantly removed from man would be used for xenografts, such as pigs instead of non-human primates. However, it is not clear that propensity to disease varies directly with phylogenetic proximity (Chapman, p.69). A persistent hepatitis E virus has been found in pigs (Chapman, p.69). In any event, xenogeneic disease theory counters a shift away from primates by identifying examples of pig-sourced zoonoses such as the global swine flu pandemic, and paramyxovirus in Australia. Another example of why phylogenetic distance cannot be taken as any kind of assurance of safety comes from the frightening hantaviruses, which pass from rodents into humans.

The "pigs can make us sick too" argument can be countered with an agreement to only use pigs grown under known pathogen-free quarantine conditions (called SPF pigs for "specified pathogen free"), so that *none* of the viruses mentioned above are present. However, xenogeneic disease theorists raise the prospect of porcine retroviruses (Swindle, p.113). These pathogens exist in all pigs in a "virtual sense" because they are simply strings of genetic code embedded in the porcine DNA (Patience, Takeuchi and Weiss, p.282). After a pig is birthed, the retrovirus code is transcribed just like the rest of the pig's DNA, but with retroviral DNA the transcribed results are viruses instead of useful proteins. Consequently, the porcine retroviruses are also called "proviruses" because they are innocuous until they are transcribed, just like a "prodrug" is a molecule that has no effect until it is catalyzed in some way by the body. The cross-species potential of retroviruses is evidenced by the fact that "despite the phylogenetic divergence of primates, cats, and mice, gibbon ape leukaemia virus and feline leukemia virus both appear to have evolved through the cross-species transmission of an ancestral C-type murine retrovirus" (Chapman, p.69).

Porcine endogenous retroviruses (PERVs) could be eliminated only with genetic engineering of the pig's DNA, a plausible task given that transgenic animals are by definition genetically engineered to avoid hyperacute rejection (Patience, p.134). In August 2000, researchers at BioTransplant, a xenotransplantation company, announced that they had in fact bred a hybrid pig that did not pass on PERVs to human cells in culture ("PERV," p.1032). However, until the entire pig genome is known, there can be no assurance that splicing out one or more known PERVs in fact has weeded out all of them. Furthermore, there tend to be multiple copies of different kinds of PERVs in each pig genome, and there appears to be substantial variation in which and how many PERVs are present in different pigs (Stoye et al., p.73). One PERV expert, Scripps Research Institute professor Daniel Salomon, believes that in five years PERVs will be "a dead issue" because only a small number of genes are responsible for transcribing all of the different PERV alleles in which the PERV transcribing genes have been deleted ("PERV," p.1032). Once these genes are identified, pigs can be cloned.

Finally, it should be pointed out that cross-species propensity to infection appears to be a two-way street. If it is difficult or easy for an animal-type virus to infect a human, it should be similarly difficult or easy for a human-type virus to infect a xenograft. As noted by the Director of Massachusetts General's Transplantation Infectious Disease Program, Dr. Jay Fishman:

> xenogenic organs may be resistant to infection with viral pathogens of humans, including HIV (1 and 2), HTLV, hepatitis viruses, and herpes viruses – including cytomegalovirus (CMV), which has been shown in our laboratory to be unable to infect porcine cells *in vitro*. Further, human hepatitis B virus does not appear to infect baboon *in vivo*. While such protection is unlikely to be observed for all potential pathogens, it may provide a significant advantage to patients with organ failure due to viral infection (Fishman, p.73).

In summary, there is certainly a theoretical possibility for xenogeneic disease transmission. From the standpoint of theory alone, however, there appears to be no way to quantify the risk. Indeed, theory alone cannot even definitively tell us whether the risk is greater or lesser based on phylogenetic proximity to man or based on type of pathogen. It would be comforting to know that the virus that destroyed a human organ would not destroy an animal replacement organ, but even that bit of theory "is unlikely to be observed for all potential pathogens" (Fishman, p.73). Consequently, we must look to practical experience with xenogeneic transmission in the handful of xenotransplantation studies that have occurred to date for further guidance.

Practical Experience with Xenogeneic Infections

In late 1999, scientists from the UK company Imutran, working with the U.S. Centers for Disease Control and Prevention, announced the results of the first large scale study of xenogeneic viral transmission. *No* sign of PERV was found in any of the 160 human patients tested who had been treated with pig skin grafts, pig pancreatic islet cells or extracorporeal pig livers, kidneys or spleens (Klotzko, p.48). Nearly a fourth of the patients had been immunosuppressed, and were thought, as a consequence, to be at greater risk of bearing PERV. The fact that 15 percent of the patients showed evidence of circulating (harmless) pig cells lent further strength to the argument that PERVs do not survive in human serum, presumably because even after months of *in vivo* existence, the pig cells did not give rise to PERVs. This data has also been interpreted to outweigh the earlier *in vitro* studies that showed PERV could infect human serum (under very artificial conditions) (Patience, Takeuchi and Weiss, p.282), since the *in vivo* environment – which is much more hostile to viruses – is the environment in which xenografts would exist (Patience, p.134).

In a similar vein, a Swedish team has reported that none of the ten diabetic patients in whom they transplanted pig pancreatic islet cells showed any evidence of PERV infection (Groth and Breimer, p.76). More generally, there are no reports that any xenograft or xenoperfusion recipient has ever become ill from any bacteria, virus, prion or other infectious agent as a result of their exposure to any animal cells, tissues or organs (*Guidance*). Furthermore, there are no reports that any xenotransplantation patient has ever passed on to a third party any microbe that passed into their body as a result of the procedure.

Conversely, in September 1999, it was reported that a baboon liver transplanted into an HIV positive patient seven years earlier had, based upon retrospective pathology work, actually passed a baboon strain of the cytomegalovirus (CMV) into the patient. This is the first documented case of a xenogeneic infection. The scientist who discovered the xenogeneic infection noted "I think it is quite concerning that an animal virus thought to be species-specific could be transmitted" ("Baboon," http://www.cnn.com). The anti-viral drug ganciclovir appeared to have cleared the CMV from the patient's system, who died for other reasons two months after receiving the transplant. Consequently, while this case demonstrates the possibility of xenogeneic infection it does not demonstrate the possibility of xenogeneic disease. In fact, it is completely expected that xenogeneic infection would occur from non-SPF animals since even a baboon scratch can transmit an infection.

Another HIV positive patient who received a baboon xenograft, although this time bone marrow rather than a liver, avoided baboon-type CMV infection because the donor baboon was raised under medical quarantine (SPF) conditions. Approximately 98 percent of baboons not quarantined from birth are infected with a variant of CMV, although it does them no harm. In summary, there is practical experience that some microbes resident in an animal will be passed to humans along with the animal's organs. There is no evidence that such microbes will cause disease. We should expect, however, that some xenogeneic microbes will cause disease simply because some zoonotic microbes cause disease in humans without any xenotransplantation.

Scientist as Lawyer: Absence of Evidence is Not Evidence of Absence

We have seen that there is no evidence of xenogeneic disease being caused by transplanted animal tissues or cells (Vanderpool 2001, p.141). However, this has not been accepted as evidence of an absence of such a possibility (FDA 2001, p.2; *Guidance*). Consequently, the tens of thousands of pig heart valves that have been transplanted into humans, without any sign of xenogeneic disease, are distinguished on the basis that the valves are preserved in glutaraldehyde, "a process which renders them nonviable, eliminates infectious organisms and reduces immune system response" (Fox and McHale, p.53). The decades of pig insulin use by diabetics and horse estrogen used by women may be distinguished on the basis of such products being mere molecules, not vascularized organs. Indeed, while CMV is difficult to transmit even via blood transfusions from an infected person, it is invariably transmitted when a human donor organ is infected (Bronsther, p.399).

Perhaps the largest xenogeneic viral infection to occur was the exposure of millions of people in the 1950s to simian virus 40 as a result of accidental contamination of polio vaccines made in primate kidney cells (Michaels, p.1). While subclinical infection was observed, nobody became ill. Even after long-term follow-up, the cancer-causing virus did not cause any increase in the cancer rate of those infected (Bronsther, p.399). This can be taken as evidence either that xenogeneic viral infection is benign, or that the risks of xenogeneic diseases are real and that society has just been lucky up until now.

Two additional factors give rise to skepticism regarding the importance of the lack of proven xenogeneic diseases up until now: immunosuppression and viral reassortment. Xenograft recipients are likely to be at least as immunosuppressed as allograft recipients. Yet immunosuppression is an inexact science, involving "a balance between the immune suppression needed to maintain graft function and the risks of opportunistic infections and cancer posed by that level of suppression" (Chapman and Fishman, p.737). As doctors endeavor to assess the right level of immunosuppression, many patients will no doubt be excessively immunosuppressed, which results in a highly favorable environment for new infections to express themselves. These new infections may not appear until large numbers of xenotransplants have occurred. Many novel infections are seen only in immunosuppressed populations such as those being treated for cancer, HIV or allotransplantation. Hence, the limited number of immunosuppressed xenograft patients to date is one of the reasons skeptics are unwilling to accept, with regard to xenogeneic diseases, that "absence of evidence is evidence of absence" (Patience, p.134).

Immunosuppression may directly affect the biggest worry of xenotransplantation, that of retroviruses. One reason that humans traditionally have not fallen ill from PERVs may be that animal viruses are easily lysed by human complement (Stoye et al., p.72). However, a key facet of defeating hyperacute rejection is the masking of a xenograft from the recipient's complement system. This same masking may permit extended survival of PERVs, with potential disease consequences. One reason no PERVs were seen in patients with xenoperfusion of porcine hepatocytes or pancreatic islet cells may have been because those patients were not immunosuppressed, due to the ability to encapsulate the pig tissues in immuno-isolation material. A different result may occur with whole organ xenografts, which requires systemic immunosuppression. On the other hand, "with the battery of tests now available to researchers, it seems safe to say that, if a PERV infection were to occur, we have the tools to accurately identify and monitor it" (Patience, p.133).

No one can realistically expect to live in a risk-free world. For example, it would be necessary to kill all birds to eliminate the natural reservoir of the flu virus. Gnotobiotic (germ-free) environments don't exist. Indeed, it is estimated that known microbes represent only about 5 percent of all microbes (Persing, p.100). Most microbes are simply not culturable, but they nevertheless can cause disease. Society does have a reasonable right to expect that those in charge of the public health system will take all practical precautions to lower, rather than increase, the overall health burden of the community. There is plenty of room for disagreement as to whether generally available xenografts would lower society's burden of death and disability by solving the problem of end-stage organ failure, or would actually increase morbidity and mortality by introducing a new pandemic. Proponents of xenotransplantation argue that a safety margin in favor of social beneficence can be accomplished with certain novel public health measures. This chapter next explores those health measures, and assesses their public acceptability.

Mi Casa Es Su Casa? Issues of Public Health Acceptability

If the unvanquishable risk of xenogeneic disease is not to be a show-stopper for xenotransplantation, it must be because there are reasonable public health measures that can contain this risk. For example, public health management of water and sewage supplies contains the risk of typhoid from dense urban living, and public health management of the blood supply contains the risk of certain blood-borne diseases. Whether or not such measures are available for xenogeneic diseases depends upon a more precise understanding of just what exactly are the theoretical danger of such diseases. The kind of public health prophylaxes needed for a long latency, highly transmissible disease are very different (and much harder to accept) than the kind of measures needed to constrain a short-acting disease.

The worst-case theoretical danger of a xenogeneic disease is that a pathogen will slip into a human host via a xenograft, have a long latency period during which it is undiscovered and transmitted to others, and then begin causing disease. If the pathogen promptly caused disease there would be little public health danger because the xeno-procedure would be promptly modified or halted (Vanderpool 2001, p.141). If the pathogen is largely non-transmissible, or only transmissible in serum, there would be modest public health danger because xenograft recipients could be barred from blood donation and counseled against unprotected sex (J. Fox, p.258). However the combination of ready transmissibility and a long latency period creates a major public health danger, in theory, because millions of people could be infected before anyone could stop the process. With over 50 million people per year dying of infectious diseases (Meslin et al., p.205), the worst-case scenario must be taken seriously.

A worst case theoretical danger might also involve the two key elements from above (long latency; easy transmissibility) plus "stealth capability" such as taking on surface antigens from the host. But the worst case theoretical disease threat, a retrovirus (like PERVs, HIV and HCV), is not necessarily a realistic threat (Patience, p.134). Despite thousands of years of close proximity, there is no indication that pigs have passed retroviruses to humans. While we can realistically assume that certain theoretical xenogeneic disease threats are possible – such as the viruses, bacteria and prions that pass from animals to men without xenotransplantation – other theoretical threats may have a near zero likelihood of being realized. Based on the foregoing theoretical risks, the question becomes whether there are *acceptable* public health measures that can guard against:

- realistic case threats such as known viruses, bacteria and prions that cause disease in man, as well as unknown microbes of reasonably short latency;
- worst-case threats such as unknown viruses of long latency, high transmissibility and unknown symptomology occurring initially in xenotransplant patients.

If the necessary public health safeguards against xenozoonotic disease are not reasonable and acceptable to people, then people won't follow them. In that event, they can't really be safeguards. However, as will be shown below, there are safeguards that are likely to be acceptable because they pose a minimal infringement to our way of life.

The U.K. Approach

The U.K. Xenotransplantation Interim Regulatory Authority (UKXIRA) is the culmination of two previous study groups, each of which produced reports. First, in 1996, the British Ministry of Health received a report from a group it had convened a year earlier, under the Chairmanship of Professor Ian Kennedy, the Advisory Group on the Ethics of Xenotransplantation. The Report, called *Animal Tissue Into Humans* but generally known as the *Kennedy Report*, concluded that primates should not be used as source animals (Kennedy 1997). This recommendation has been adopted by all subsequent UK reviews, and was also adopted as a basic prophylactic health measure by the UKXIRA, since it stops a whole class of simian-human common viruses at the gate. This recommendation also addressed the issue of *realistic* retrovirus threats since the only zoonotic retrovirus believed to be responsible for a human disease is the Simian Immunodeficiency Virus (SIV), the evolutionary precursor to HIV. Unaddressed, however, is the worst-case scenario of a disease-causing porcine retrovirus.

Also in 1996, the private Nuffield Council on Bioethics issued a report that similarly barred primates as xenograft sources, but expressly blessed the use of pigs as organ sources subject to the implementation of an appropriate governmental regime to ensure SPF environments, expansive patient surveillance procedures, and ethically appropriate protocols (Nuffield, p.112). The Xenotransplantation Interim Regulatory Authority was formed as proposed by the

Kennedy and Nuffield Reports, and is operating according to guidelines consistent with those reports ("Guidance").

In October 1999, the United Kingdom became the first country in the world to adopt a formal regime of public health prophylaxes against xenogeneic diseases. These rules were adopted by the Xenotransplantation Interim Regulatory Authority. In particular, the new regulations advised patients receiving xenografts to consent to "life-long surveillance and agree never to have children" (Rogers, p.7). The UKXIRA has left it to sponsors of xenotransplantation trials to propose specific life-long surveillance protocols. As of November 2000, three such proposals had been submitted to UKXIRA. Although two of the three were authorized, the sponsors have not yet proceeded to clinical trials ("Third Annual," p.12). While the child-bearing restriction may appear harsh, it will not be perceived that way if xenotransplant teams explain in the informed consent process that this is necessary to avoid endangering newborns with a congenital xenovirus. Furthermore, there is always the option of adoption and, for men, pre-transplantation storage of semen for post-transplant *in vitro* fertilization, if desired. Consequently, to date, the UK safeguards are reasonable and likely to be complied with. This means that they are not illusory safeguards.

The U.S. Approach

The FDA approached xenotransplantation regulation exactly as it would if it had safety concerns with any new drug or treatment. It placed a clinical hold on it until it was reasonably assured that studies could be carried out safely. The industry, clinicians and patients accepted the public health measures asked for by the FDA without objection. The FDA dealt with a worst-case threat (PERV retroviruses), but treated it like a realistic threat (if it is not seen in an assay post-transplant, then there is no reason to stop the trial). The FDA was no more likely to wait decades to see if some worst-case scenario such as a latent, highly transmissible virus was going to manifest itself, than it would be willing to hold-up new drug approvals for decades to see if some untoward side effect appeared in a new mass market drug. In the FDA's view, if a xenograft does not appear infectious, the reasonable course appears to be to conduct very careful monitoring for signs of infectivity, but otherwise to proceed with development (Vanderpool 2001, p.142). Similarly, if a new drug does not appear to be unsafe, the reasonable course is to stay alert to signs of danger, but to otherwise proceed with commercialization.

In February 2001, the FDA issued a *Draft Guidance* document for industry concerning xenotransplantation activities. This document did not change the FDA's approach, but went into much greater detail regarding how to minimize the risks of xenogeneic disease by specifying rigorous source animal selection criteria (FDA 2001, p.16). The document also provided specific instructions as to its expectations for long-term biomonitoring of xenograft patients and archiving of biosamples from them to minimize the risk that any xenogeneic disease would be widely transmitted before it was identified (FDA 2001, p.50). Finally, the FDA became quite specific regarding the high level of sensitivity to xenogeneic infectious agents that it expected from assays used in xenotransplantation protocols (FDA 2001, p.25).

Clearly it will be necessary to rely on surveillance of the post-transplant population to ensure that no latent infections are brewing in human society. While the main pillar of public health prophylaxes against xenogeneic diseases is the use of SPF pigs consistent with animal welfare rules, there will still be a need for a long-term if not life-long patient surveillance regimen adequate to deal with the risk of infectious disease transmission from pigs (Institute of Medicine 1996, p.56). Are there surveillance regimens that are acceptable for dealing with non-latent risks? With latent risks?

Stasi Medicine? – How Surveillance Can Coexist with Human Rights

One of the more rigorous efforts to clearly definitize the word "right" is the schema adopted by Wesley Hohfeld, in the early 20th century, born of his own frustration with the legal profession's failure to recognize that "chameleon-hued words are a peril both to clear thought and to lucid expression" (Hohfeld, p.35). Hohfeld taught that "right" is the correlative of "duty" and the opposite of "no-right", whereas "privilege" is the correlative of "no-right" and the opposite of "duty" (Hohfeld, pp.36-38). Hohfield offers up "claim" as a synonym for right, noting that a "right" or a "claim" has meaning in the sense of its correlate concept of "duty." Hence, if a patient has the right to make an autonomous decision regarding the refusal of therapeutic treatment, then there must be a reciprocal duty on the part of the practitioner to respect that right. Defining rights in this way is consistent with many ordinary uses of the term (e.g. the right to vote, to exercise free speech, and to own and control private property). There can be no question that one of the defining features of a democratic society is the priority that is placed on respect for individual rights defined in this way.

Despite the importance of individual rights-as-claims, there are also accepted limitations on such rights. For example, individuals are permitted to exercise control over their private property to the degree that they do not use it to threaten the health and safety of others. Were this to be so, their control – if not their property – would be taken from them. In the sphere of health care, similar examples also hold. The power of quarantine is an example of a draconian power granted to health officials that allows them to restrict personal autonomy. Thus any society that embraces the moral importance of human rights ordinarily does so by balancing the equities of personal autonomy and public health benefits. Xenotransplantation is no different.

With a conception of autonomy – including informed consent – in mind, the issue that must be adversed head-on is the possibility of reconciling the necessity for effective surveillance, as described above, with legitimate constraints on autonomy. There can be no question that a dramatic threat is indeed potentially posed by the type of surveillance widely regarded as required to avert a xenogeneic pandemic.

It seems likely that submission to lifelong biopsy and blood sampling would be acceptable to transplant recipients because that kind of invasive monitoring is standard medical practice, even for allotransplant patients today. The FDA proposes a not unduly burdensome biosampling frequency for patients and "persons with whom recipients repeatedly engage in activities that could result in intimate exchange of body fluids" (*Draft Guidance*, para. VIII.F.4). The proposed schedule calls for blood, plasma and urine samples "(a) prior to xenotransplantation (two samples, one month apart), (b) at the time of transplantation, (c) in the immediate post-transplant period, (d) at one month and six months after transplant, (e) annually for the first two years, and (f) every five years subsequently" (*Draft Guidance*, para. VIII.F.3.c.i). The Organisation for Economic Co-operation and Development (OECD) has further amplified what it considers to be key components of an internationally-obligatory xenotransplant patient surveillance program:

> The potential for animal microbial agents to be pathogenic in the human recipient following xenotransplantation and to be transmissible to others alters the traditional understanding of informed consent, since it would involve not only the subject but *also close contacts and ultimately the community*. Informed consent in xenotransplantation is also complicated by the potential requirement of *strict* postoperative monitoring and by:
>
> - the state of uncertainty;
> - the need for lifelong surveillance and *contact monitoring*;
> - the potential of risks for contacts, and including health-care workers.
>
> (*Xenotransplantation*, p.80) (emphasis added).

The OECD does not explain what it means by contact monitoring, but it may include asking contacts of the patient whether the patient has complied with prohibitions against exchanging bodily fluids ("Emerging," para. 3.4), and asking contacts of the patient to submit themselves to blood tests for xenogeneic infections. These conditions are also likely to be acceptable to patients facing death: the family of the patient with AIDS who received a baboon marrow transplant agreed to be monitored in these ways, and the patient agreed to refrain from unprotected sex. But are the conditions acceptable to co-workers, neighbors, or friends? How can informal "contacts" of the patient be placed under biosurveillance without their consent?

In addition to contact monitoring, it may be necessary to engage in some amount of large-scale population surveillance for emerging xenogeneic diseases, especially as xenotransplantation becomes more widespread or if xenogeneic infections are discovered. Would not such surveillance run into strong objections based on violation of autonomy, and thereby present a stumbling block to any implementation of xenotransplantation? Might this especially be the case for international xenotransplantation monitoring, as noted by Eugene Brody in *Biomedical Technology and Human Rights* [9]:

> The process of introducing new biomedical technology and its trained operators from a complex individualistic culture into a less complex collectivist community cannot leave the community unchanged. The symbolic and interactional context of life which contributes to any individual's sense of meaning and worth is altered. Further, those who introduce and manage the technology are figures of power, often perceived as outstripping the local healers. This may place the rights, privileges and obligations of the entire community at risk. Under these circumstances an authentic process of informed consent for treatment with the new devices or procedures may be impossible.

Informed consent turns out not to be an obstacle to xenotransplantation. Where it is particularly important (for the ongoing bio-monitoring of a patient and their contacts) it is readily obtainable through face-to-face meetings. Of course, this presupposes that those obtaining consent have the training and communication skills in order to effectively communicate with those agreeing to be biosurveillance subjects and that such subjects have the levels of understanding required to make whatever consent that is given fully informed. To the degree that both of these conditions are met, consent is readily obtainable through appropriate face-to-face meetings and only its life-long non-cancellability raises new moral issues. As a practical matter, a xenograft recipient or their intimate contacts should not have the right to withdraw their consent to ongoing bio-monitoring unless and until it is scientifically agreed that the xenotransplant, which was received on the basis of such consent, poses no significant public risk. Equally, it may be the case that after a certain point, it will be scientifically agreed that surveillance can take a minimal profile (e.g. epidemiological sampling). In this case, individuals who had consented to surveillance in return for a xenograft for themselves or their relatives would be relieved of their more stringent original obligations. In any case, the law has been clear for a century or more that it is acceptable to withdraw respect from autonomy rights in the face of circumstances where there is wide agreement that respecting them potentially undermines the health and safety of others – including, in the U.S., mandatory vaccination (*Jacobson v. Massachusetts*, 197 U.S. 11, 25-27 (1905)). Given the dramatic threat to public health potentially posed by xenotransplantation, and the minimal inconvenience of biomonitoring, it is not unreasonable to require the modest impingement on autonomy of non-cancellability of informed consent to bio-monitoring.

Where informed consent is difficult to obtain, such as in support of community-wide biosurveillance for xenozoonotic organisms, it is not morally required provided that the results of the research are not traceable back to an individual. Finally, if there is a desire to trace the results of community-wide surveillance back to infected individuals, then adequate effort and resources must be invested in obtaining informed consent and in protecting the confidentiality of the obtained information. These points are expanded upon below.

Consent, Informed or Presumed?

The bioethical precept of autonomy and the basic human right – stated in the Nuremberg Code and the Helsinki Declaration – to consent prior to being made a research subject, are very important principles. However, they are not absolute. An important degree of flexibility can be seen in how the clinically-driven Helsinki Declaration varies from the judicially-written Nuremberg Code.

More concretely, the Siracusa Principles, adopted in 1999, are considered by the United Nations as a checklist for restricting even important human rights, excluding a few absolute rights such as freedom from torture or slavery, but including the right to be free of research protocols absent informed consent:

> Interference with most rights can be legitimately justified as necessary under narrowly defined circumstances in many situations relevant to public health. Limitations on rights, however, are considered a serious issue under international human rights law, regardless of the apparent importance of the public good involved. When a government limits the exercise or enjoyment of a right, this action must be taken only as a last resort and will only be considered legitimate if the following criteria are met:
>
> 1. The restriction is provided for and carried out in accordance with the law;
> 2. The restriction is in the interest of a legitimate objective of general interest;
> 3. The restriction is strictly necessary in a democratic society to achieve the objective;
> 4. There are no less intrusive and restrictive means available to reach the same goal; and
> 5. The restriction is not imposed arbitrarily, i.e., in an unreasonable or otherwise discriminatory manner (Gruskin and Tarantola).

When a xenograft recipient develops a possible infectious syndrome (a near certainty among any transplant recipient), one expert proposes the following burdensome but probably bearable protocol:

> the patient must be admitted to the transplant center (not an outlying hospital) and placed on contact precautions, with respiratory isolation in a neutral or negative pressure environment . . . . All patient contacts are governed by universal precautions with gown, gloves, masks and shoe covers. In addition to routine microbiologic samples (blood, sputum, urine, stools) or tissue biopsies, sera and leukocytes are obtained for immediate testing and also stored for future study . . . . Quarantine would be maintained until a specific microbiologic diagnosis is achieved. Serologic assays might be repeated at monthly intervals. Cultures and serologies should also be obtained on family and sexual contacts (A. Fishman, p.61).

If the public health measures considered adequate to guard against even latent infections are simply life-long monitoring of the patient and their contacts, modest lifestyle restrictions and limited, short-term quarantine until illnesses are diagnosed, then informed consent is unlikely to present a barrier to the implementation of xenotransplantation (Vanderpool 2001, p.141). Unlike the emotion-driven public opposition that suppresses commerce in human organs and compulsory cadaveric transplants, there is little emotive basis for public opposition to xenotransplant safeguards. The revulsion that most people feel toward human organ sales simply does not exist with regard to mandatory family cooperation with a patient's medical follow-up protocol, i.e. biosurveillance. Similarly, religious concepts about the dead and their organs are not evident when talking about reasonable steps to prevent xenodisease transmission.

The reasonableness of public health safeguards against xenodisease withstands even the inability of the consenters to withdraw their initial informed consent. The reasons for this are:

- Medical authorities *are complying* with bioethical or human rights norms by constructing their xenotransplantation protocols to include informed consent from the patient as well as a described set of patient intimate contacts, provided that an impartial, review group confirms the reasonableness of the protocol (Weijer, p.354). If either the patient or their intimate contacts refuse to sign the informed consent form, then the medical authorities are under no obligation to provide the xenotransplantation procedure. Indeed, they should not (*Third Annual*, para. 5.8-10).

- If the patient or their contacts attempt to *withdraw* their consent after xenotransplantation, they can be reminded of their obligations to the community. If they are not presenting an infectious disease threat to the community, increasingly persuasive measures up through coercion should be adopted to obtain their compliance with their informed consent (Daar, "Choosing," p.165). The usual autonomy right to rescind informed consent is circumscribed with xenotransplantation because of the potential risk of a xenogeneic pandemic. However, if the xenograft recipients or their contacts do present an infectious disease threat to the community, they may be quarantined regardless of informed consent because autonomy is not an absolute right and would in this case be trumped by public health concerns (subject to the Siracusa Principles checklist set forth above).

Consents given by the patient and their intimate contacts – such as promising to use a barrier to prevent the exchange of fluids during sex – may be "unenforceable by law . . . appropriate patient selection is therefore crucial" (*Third Annual*, para. 5.10). One way to help ensure appropriate patient selection is by requiring patients (and their intimate contacts) to sign "Ulysses contracts." These are enduring, irrevocable advance directives that authorize third parties, by force if necessary, to ensure the contractor's compliance with post-xenotransplantation obligations (Daar, "Choosing," p.165). As is the case with allotransplantation, careful socio-psychological pre-screening, education and counseling is needed to minimize the number of patients (and patient contacts for xenotransplantation) that become lost to follow-up or who are otherwise non-compliant with their agreed-upon obligations (*Draft Guidance*, para. VIII.D). Indeed, the education and counseling process may need to be long to help remind xenograft recipients and their contacts of the moral importance of their obligations, and to thereby ensure the highest possible rate of follow-up compliance.

Ethnographic studies of xenograft recipients have shown them to be quite willing to put up with all manner of burdens and risks in order to achieve their overarching desire to remain alive (Lundin, p.151). In addition, patients will be very much less likely to wish to withdraw their informed consent if the bio-monitoring regime is constructed consistently with respect for human rights, as has been nicely outlined by the WHO in its guidance on xenotransplantation:

> every effort will be made to protect recipients from the initiation or continuation of unreasonable measures. Review boards with expertise in xenotransplantation, infectious diseases, public health principles, bioethics, and civil rights should be established to decide when such measures are necessary and how long they should be practiced. Review boards should be empowered to resolve disputes generated from the initiation and maintenance of infectious disease assessment and containment measures. Recipients should be informed about the function of these boards and how to access them expeditiously. Follow-up infectious disease assessment and containment procedures must be consistent with basic human rights principles (WHO 1998, para. 7.0).

The late Jonathan Mann championed the importance of conflating public health and human rights, noting that "human rights violations have health impacts, that is, adverse effects on physical, mental, and social well-being" (Mann 1999, p.445). He and others have documented that:

> discrimination toward HIV-infected people and people with AIDS is counterproductive. Specifically, when people found to be infected were deprived of employment, education, or ability to marry and travel, participation in prevention programs diminished. Thus, recent attention has been directed to a negotiation process for optimizing both the achievement of complementary public health goals and respect for human rights norms (Mann 1999, p.445).

Years before Dr. Mann's observations, around 1970, a similar situation was played out involving newly available hepatitis B antigen testing. At first, there was some movement in the direction of identifying, and stigmatizing, all those who tested positive. However, thanks to efforts of people, such as Baruch Blumberg, the developer of the test, that thinking was shown to be flawed (Blumberg, "Bioethical," p.852). He pointed out that the public health benefit of excluding blood that tested positive from the transfusion pool could be accomplished anonymously. To identify carriers when there was no treatment for the virus presented a real harm to the carrier (discrimination), but only a tenuous and unclear benefit to the public (possible avoidance of infection with a generally latent virus). In Dr. Mann's matrix, violating the human rights of HBV carriers has adverse health effects on both the individual and on the entire public health system, which is undermined by reactive public noncompliance with it. The ideal solution would be to immunize everyone against HBV, as that would ensure a benefit to everyone without stigmatization to anyone (this is now possible, but expensive). Alternatively, if the plan is that only contacts of a carrier are to be vaccinated, such a plan will only work, and be ethical, if the carrier and his or her contacts are protected from stigmatization.

Adherence to the WHO guidelines on xenotransplantation would certainly help to ensure a high degree of voluntary compliance with recipient and contact life-long informed consent, because there would be little fear of unjust consequences. However, in the final analysis, neither withdrawal of informed consent nor the shield of confidentiality will protect an intimate contact of a xenograft recipient with a transmissible xenogeneic disease from the long arm of public health.

One ambiguous issue at the nexus of xenotransplantation and consent involves the scope of the term "contacts." If contacts are "intimate contacts," then they are readily identifiable and may be handled as set forth above, consistently with conventional interpretations of informed consent. But what if contacts include "casual contacts" – co-workers, co-commuters, and co-diners? This ever-increasing assortment of people with whom a xenograft recipient may share personal space cannot sensibly be covered under any kind of written informed consent document. This population of "casual contacts" provides a good example of a situation in which the medical ethics concept of informed consent does not really fit with public health realities. A reasonable implementation of "casual contact" biosurveillance for xenogeneic infection might involve requiring, on a random basis, xenogeneic blood tests from those receiving public health care. The infringement on autonomy would be rendered *de minimis* if mechanisms ensured anonymity, and yet that condition would not necessarily diminish the value of the epidemiological research. While there is an infringement of autonomy, it is not a material infringement and it is done to secure greater health care for all.

Community Consent

In addition to relying on the likely voluntary cooperation of a patient's intimate contacts, and anonymous random-checking of the community, there is also the concept of community consent. Notwithstanding the ability of public health agencies to address realistic and even worst-case xenogeneic risks by mandating biomonitoring of those at risk and that only SPF pig organs be used, it has been argued that no extent of prophylactic measures are adequate for the risks of xenogeneic diseases *without* express *community* consent (Bach, p.66). The contrary view is that neither a referendum nor a precipitous decision is necessary because the bioethical requirement of informed consent applies to the patient, not third parties like "the public." In this view, acceptable public health prophylactic measures can adequately ensure that the public is not a *de facto* experimental subject.

There is international bioethical recognition of the concept of community consent. The *International Guidelines for Ethical Review of Epidemiological Studies* provide that:

> When it is not possible to request informed consent from every individual to be studied, the agreement of a representative of a community or group may be sought, but the representative should be chosen according to the nature, traditions and political philosophy of the community or group . . . . However, the refusal of individuals to participate in a study has to be respected: a leader may express agreement on behalf of a community, but an individual's refusal of personal participation is binding (CIOMS, p.12).

In the case of xenotransplantation, when a representative government decides (either via legislation or referendum) to authorize the procedure within its jurisdiction, it can consent to biosurveillance on behalf of the population it represents because it is not possible to seek the informed consent of every person who may have contact with a xenograft recipient. However, such consent cannot morally include the identification of individuals, without their individual informed consent:

> If we cannot afford to conduct medical research so that the autonomy of participants really is respected then the research should not be done. Otherwise, we risk pretending that informed consent has been obtained because certain rituals have been performed (e.g. the signing of a piece of paper). To rest content with such gestures – to equate them with an acceptable level of informed consent in either research of non-experimental therapy – remains a breach of human rights and an offence against human dignity (Doyal, "The Moral," p.317).

The *International Guidelines for Ethical Review of Epidemiological Studies* do provide individuals under community consent conditions with the right to opt out of research. Individuals can refuse to be biosampled for xenogeneic infections, even if there has been community consent. However, should such individuals nevertheless evidence frank disease, the principle of autonomy is trumped by the rights of everyone else not to be exposed to infectious disease – the recalcitrant individuals may be quarantined.

While it is clear that such biosurveillance and monitoring will not absolutely prevent a latent, highly transmissible disease from causing an epidemic, the monitoring would significantly reduce the likelihood of even this worst-case possibility by:

- constantly looking for new infectious agents in patients and contacts serum, and thus probably finding them sooner rather than later (Chapman and Fishman, p.739); and,
- enabling a prompt quarantine of at least the patients and their known contacts in the event of a worst case scenario.

By comparison with the only known zoonotic latent retrovirus infection, HIV:

- no one was looking for HIV until it had already caused odd diseases;
- even after HIV was found, little was done in the public health arena due to its stigmatization with homosexuality and injection drug use;
- there remains no program of infected patient monitoring except in the case of a few pathological "disease vector" individuals.

Furthermore, there are tools available today to discover latent infectious organisms that were not available when AIDS broke out in the early 1980s. These tools are known as broad-range (or "consensus") polymerase chain reaction (PCR) and representational difference analysis (RDA) (Patience, p.133). Each of these techniques permits the identification of novel infectious agents as to which there are no pre-existing assays or screening tests (Persing, p.750). With these new technologies, and with periodic blood tests, it can be reasonably expected that novel pathogens will be detected in the serum of a xenograft recipient prior to, or soon after, the onset or initial transmission of a xenogeneic disease (Patience, p.133). Indeed the new consensus PCR and RDA technologies are expected to "contribute to a tremendous expansion of knowledge regarding the etiologic basis of many human diseases" (Persing, p.750). This pathogen-scanning capability is especially important in the transplant context – be it allotransplant or xenotransplant – because immunosuppression of the recipient often makes it more difficult to detect clinical symptoms of illness.

Life Trumps Autonomy?

A final set of facts to explore surrounds the conduct of biosurveillance in which the results are traceable back to an individual. For example, to further reduce the risk of a delayed pandemic break-out of a latent, infectious retrovirus, society may decide that biosurveillance results need to be linkable to individuals. Such information could be useful in rapidly identifying those persons who should take precautions against further transmission or who could benefit from any anti-viral medications that might be developed. As explained above, all such situations morally require informed consent. Consequently, some individuals will never agree to be biosampled for xenogeneic diseases, while others will agree readily, perhaps in connection with routine medical care or blood donations. In addition, consenters will certainly have an expectation of confidentiality.

The best solution to the tension between the human rights and the health care aspects of xenotransplantation is to implement population-based biosurveillance only on a *non-traceable, random sampling basis*. In this way society gains the benefit of understanding the prevalence, if any, of xenogeneic viruses, without risking infringement of the autonomy of its members. The downside of this approach – losing more rapid identification of persons infected with a xenogeneic virus – is speculative because it is not expected that there will be *casually* transmissible xenogeneic infections, and if there are, then locating only those who have been bio-sampled will make little difference in the spread of the infection. The upside of the blinded approach to biosurveillance is concrete – an additional item of confidential information or biosample is not obtained from autonomous members of society.

The foregoing analysis of technical risks from xenotransplantation has highlighted the dilemma between private and public interests engendered by this potential therapeutic modality. The risks are uncertain, unquantifiable and, in light of the long latency period for retroviruses, possibly unknowable within a reasonable policymaking timeframe. Yet, any policy position taken effectively presumes a risk profile.

If the public is asked to give its "informed consent" there is a presumption that the public would be an experimental subject, that is, there is a meaningful risk of xenogeneic disease. If the public is not asked to give its "informed consent" there is a presumption that the risk to the public can be rendered *de minimis* via acceptable public health measures – which themselves impinge upon the autonomy of third persons such as the patient's contacts. There still does not appear to be any way to tell whether the risk is, in fact, meaningful or meaningless.

Much of the tension between informed consent and xenotransplantation arises from the bifurcation of medicine and public health. The values of medicine are expressed in terms of "ethics", whereas in public health:

> the usefulness of the language and structure of ethics as we know it today has been questioned. Given its population focus and its interest in the underlying conditions upon which health is predicated (and that these major determinants of health status are societal in nature), it seems evident that a framework that expresses fundamental values in societal terms, and a vocabulary of values that links directly with societal structure and function, may be better adapted to the work of public health than a more individually oriented ethical framework. For this reason, modern human rights, precisely because they were initially developed entirely outside the health domain and seek to articulate the societal preconditions

> for human well-being, seem a far more useful framework, vocabulary, and form of guidance for public health efforts (Mann, pp.445-46).

In order to use human rights as the ethical value set for public health, Mann argues that public health needs to "divest itself of its biomedical conceptual foundation" and to focus on derogations of dignity and other oppressive social conditions as the targets of the public health sector's efforts. In this worldview, the key issues for containing the risks of xenogeneic disease are not *only* whether the animals are "clean" and some set of people consented to biosurveillance for those risks. Instead, for public health, of equal, if not paramount, importance should be the issue of whether the patients, contacts and susceptible populations are able to combat those risks should they occur. Exercising autonomy is very important, but improving the lives of the people who may be hit hardest by a xenogeneic virus is "job number one."

Conclusion

Xenotransplantation presents a clear conflict between private and public interests in biomedical technology. No existing rules of bioethics can tell us whether to go or to stop because the risk is unassessable. We are left with the rather absurd result that, within Europe alone, the UK says "go" while the Swiss say "stop." The absurdity is heightened by the ability of a Swiss patient to fly to the UK for a procedure, by a UK patient to travel to Switzerland for leisure, and by the hypothesized xenogeneic viruses – whether they be harmless or harmful – to travel virtually anywhere, and possibly replicate.

However, it is possible for both private and public constituencies to accept the risks of xenotransplantation, consistently with the basic human right of autonomy. This right is ordinarily implemented in medicine as the obligation to obtain the informed consent of an experimental subject, and it is certainly obligatory for a xenograft recipient. But the right is not absolute. Public health considerations can trump the right to the extent it is necessary to contain xenogeneic disease in the general population. In addition, there are globally acceptable mechanisms for obtaining community consent. Indeed, such community consent is likely to be a key aspect of any resolution of the private/public conflict over xenotransplantation. The WHO summarized the situation well when it concluded that:

> Despite the concerns and difficulties listed above, xenotransplantation could have the potential for relatively safe implementation. Since we do not have a complete understanding of all potentially pertinent infectious agents, a complete elimination of risk for both the individual recipient and for the general population will probably not be achievable. If precautions are taken, however, the risks could be reduced to that which may be considered acceptable and outweighed by the benefits of the technology (WHO 1998, para. 6.0).

As a practical matter, only those patients that contractually obligate themselves and persuade their intimate contacts to contract themselves, via the informed consent process, to comply with lifelong biosurveillance will be permitted access to xenografts. Until such time that there is a scientific consensus regarding the safety to public health of xenografts, one will not have a right to withdraw from such biosurveillance, just as one does not have a right to publicly transmit a frankly expressed serious disease. No doubt, there will be exceptions that fall through the cracks of such a scheme. However, the difficult-to-transmit, long-latency diseases that worry epidemiologists do not become pandemic through a few exceptions. Consequently, the less-than-perfect nature of mandatory biosurveillance does not diminish its ability to adequately address the xenozoonotic epidemic risks of xenotransplantation.

In addition to the need to manage with precautionary steps the theorized but unproven xenogeneic disease risks of xenotransplantation, there are other sorts of risks posed by the procedure. These "non-technological" risks include theological, philosophical, and psychological considerations of using animal organs to extend human life. The next chapter analyzes whether any of these risks present insurmountable obstacles to the advent of xenotransplantation.

Chapter IV

Of Pigs and Men: Issues of Speciesism and Chimerism

In previous chapters we saw that the "organ gap" is most feasibly solved with xenografts, subject to an assessment of the public's willingness to accept xenotransplantation. From a scientific perspective, the possibility of xenogeneic disease is the most formidable risk to public acceptance of xenotransplantation. Chapter III showed that managing this risk would require extensions of standard public health measures, including a comprehensive surveillance program of the xenorecipient and of those with whom they might have infectious contact. Indeed, such measures are already in the process of being implemented in the United Kingdom and the United States. It is the objective of this chapter, however, to assess whether there are *other* types of harm caused by xenotransplantation that could impede its development. These other types of harm are non-scientific in nature, being grounded in "social concerns" for animal well-being or human-animal chimerism.

Introduction

A 1999 U.K. poll published in the *The Times* noted that transplants of organs into humans from animal donors was supported by only 44 percent of the sample and opposed by 42 percent (Ahuja, p.36). These numbers tilted slightly to 50 percent and 39 percent, respectively, if the question was qualified by saying that the xenograft was "necessary to achieve a permanent cure for Alzheimer's disease" (Ahuja, p.36). Both sets of responses compared poorly with the poll's 90 percent acceptance rate of transplants of organs into humans from human donors, and a sobering 71 percent of the sample opposed genetic modification of animals (unless the reason was for a cure for Alzheimer's, in which case 54 percent were opposed). On the other hand, a poll taken in the U.S. indicated that 75 percent of the public would use a xenograft for a family member if a human organ was unavailable ("Poll," p.315). Other polling data suggests that if the public thought xenotransplantation was as successful as allotransplantation, then both procedures would have similar approval rates (Cassileth et al., p.148).

More recent polling data shows a growing trend toward acceptance of xenotransplantation. A two-year study of 16,500 members of the European Union, surveyed across 15 member states, found evidence of growing acceptance and knowledge of xenotransplantation (Europeans and Biotechnology, p.13). Support of xenotransplantation and tolerance for risk increased over the two periods in which the survey was administered, from 1996 to 2002. Similarly, opposition to the technology decreased significantly over that time. Interestingly, support for xenotransplantation grew, while skepticism for other technologies, such as genetically modified (GM) foods and crops, which started off at the same level of approval, saw a marked increase.

It is wise to remember that other potential solutions to the organ shortage, such as an "organ draft" or an "organ market," are unavailable due to the non-scientific "social factor" of the public's virulent distaste for such activities. Consequently, serious attention needs to be given to non-science-based concerns, such as "animal rights" and "natural order of things." Because such claims are not based on science, they can be more difficult to overcome than the widely recognized concerns regarding new zoonotic diseases (Turville-Heitz, p.32).

Are All Animals Created Equal?

As previously described, pigs are the only animals under serious consideration as xenograft sources. It would not be practical to raise non-human primates in the quantity needed to address the organ gap (although baboons have been the favored "proof of concept" animals in the limited xenotransplant studies conducted to date). Among other mammals, porcine organs are also uniquely well size-matched to human needs. An examination of animal interests in xenotransplantation can reasonably focus on the interests of pig.

What obligations do or should humans have in providing for animal welfare? From the time of Aristotle, through St. Thomas Aquinas, and to the current time, there has been agreement upon a categorization of life into plants, animals and humans (which are of course also animals). There has been little agreement as to whether there is a human duty to provide for animal welfare in general. Some have argued that there is no such duty since animals are more like plants than like man (Leahy, p.85). Others have contended that there is a human duty born of Christian charity and benevolence doctrine to avoid what appears as unnecessary animal suffering (Linzey, p.181). Utilitarian liberationists claim there is a duty to treat clearly sentient animals like similarly situated people because these animals are more like men than plants (Singer, p.61). And radicals assert that animals have an "inherent right" to autonomy as to which humans have no moral right to interfere, absent self-defense. Clearly a generally agreed-upon moral theory does not exist that unambiguously guides human behavior toward animals.

We Feel Your Pain

Philosophers have long argued over whether non-human animals have interests, or are mere automatons without any interests (like inanimate objects). In the late 18th century Jeremy Bentham recognized the ability of an animal to suffer as the benchmark of whether it had interests that could be impugned (Bentham 1960, p.411). Over a century earlier, Descartes denied the possibility of animal interests by deeming them mere *automata*, a view which gained further credence a century later with the rise of empirical behaviorism and the awarding of the Nobel Prize to animal experimentalist Pavlov. Critics of animal interests attribute the apparent suffering of animals to human perceptions of their reflex reactions, such as the use by humans of anthropomorphic "language-games" to construct animal "pain" out of mere neuromuscular animal reflexes (Leahy, p.125; Wittgenstein, p.23). Successors to Jeremy Bentham, however, counter that:

> Some nonhuman animals appear to be rational and self-conscious beings, conceiving themselves as distinct beings with a past and a future. When this is so, or *to the best of our knowledge may be so*, the case against killing is strong, as strong as the case against killing permanently defective human beings at a similar mental level (Singer, *Practical*, 103) (emphasis added).

The italicized words form the Rubicon between those who believe pigs and other animals have interests and those who believe they do not. There is no objective, scientific means of determining whether or not nonhuman animals are "self-conscious beings." Consequently, advocates of animal interests say we should *err on the side of caution*, and if the animal appears to be rational and self-conscious, then we should treat it as similarly situated humans would be treated. Debunkers of animal interests claim the likelihood of animal self-consciousness is so remote that it would be absurd and counter-utilitarian to accord their well-being any consideration beyond what is necessary to assuage human squeamishness.

Agreeing to Disagree

This chapter will show that common ground *can be* established if the focus of debate is shifted from "whether pigs are self-conscious beings" to "whether domesticated animals are a form of life that deserves respect." It will be shown that virtually everyone believes that animals such as pigs are entitled to a measure of respect – that, for example, it is wrong to sadistically torture them, or to burn them alive. Whether that respect permits sacrificing pigs for xenografts depends upon whether such sacrifice is consistent with generally accepted hierarchies of moral value. Under such hierarchies avoidance of life-threatening pain and suffering in a self-conscious being, such as a human, trumps avoidance of death to a being that is not known to be self-conscious, such as a pig – especially if the death is carried out painlessly, and with respect shown to the animal. In other words, only the most extreme advocates of animal rights would disagree that an animal could be painlessly killed, without any awareness of its impending death, to save the life of a fully cognizant human.

The consensus underlying the hierarchy of moral value is not that humans are "better than" animals; instead, according respect to life implies a need for greater deference to clearly self-conscious life than to clearly sentient but only ambiguously self-conscious life. Self-conscious life is tender, since self-awareness makes one fear the death and disability that can accompany disease. Hence it is our respect for life that leads us to sacrifice pigs to prolong human life, just as it is our respect for life that obligates us to take great care that porcine organ donors are treated kindly, and not frightened or caused pain. The hierarchy of moral value is not "speciesist." Human suffering trumps painless, unaware animal death only because the human happens to be self-conscious of the suffering (not because s/he happens to be human), and self-conscious suffering is a worse insult to the sanctity of life than an unaware death for the purpose of saving a life.

However, this summary of the argument to be pursued will remain no more than an abstraction without some examination and evaluation of the arguments of the chief proponents. As will be shown, the wide gulf between those who support and oppose animal experimentation may suggest the impossibility of a coherent compromise; the argument here will demonstrate that one is possible.

Singer: Weigh Animals Like Humans

Peter Singer expounded a general theory of animal rights in his landmark volume, *Animal Liberation*. In this volume, Singer grafted the popular philosophical paradigm of utilitarianism onto the evolving conclusion of animal behavior studies that primates and other higher mammals display many facets of sentience. These include the ability to experience pleasure, pain and suffering – and possibly self-consciousness – the ability to reflect on oneself as part of the larger world in both time and space. Consequently, argued Singer, the quest of utilitarian reasoning, to authorize those actions that bring the best results to the greatest numbers, should apply not only with regard to numbers of humans, but with regard to numbers of animals as well, at least sentient, possibly self-conscious animals. Singer's theory requires society to balance the interests of animals equally with those of humans in setting policy. Under this theory vegetarianism would be mandatory because animals are better off not being eaten and since humans won't die for lack of meat. All other things being equal, Singer's theory would proscribe the sacrifice of an animal life for a human life, since he values the lives commensurately.

Singer's theory is plagued by a systematic inconsistency – his insistence on treating fundamentally dissimilar beings in a similar fashion. For example, while he uses the capacity to feel pain as a species' membership pass into utilitarian policymaking, he struggles over the very different kinds of pain that exist in the animal kingdom. He does not even know how many species should be included because he does not know how far the experience of pain goes down the evolutionary ladder, and he is even more clueless as to the dispersion of self-consciousness across the species. He believes there are varying levels of self-consciousness among higher animal species, but his theory cannot accommodate the varying sensitivities of these species without jettisoning the fundamental premise of equal treatment for humans and animals. Singer hoped to offer a theory to treat similar things (those beings that suffer pain) similarly. Instead, he proposes to treat dissimilar things (beings who suffer and experience very different kinds of pain) similarly. The net result is unlikely to offer the greatest good for the greatest number because dissimilar units (beings) cannot be rationally combined with equal weight in a utilitarian calculus.

Another problem with Singer is that he effectively gives to animals "rights" from human interference with their well-being without assigning the animals any corresponding "duties" to obey laws, pay taxes, and so on. Singer defends himself on this charge by alleging that the animals are no differently situated than human mental defectives who also enjoy rights without corresponding duties. Singer ignores, however, that humans have reduced sets of rights in proportion to their ability to act in accord with obligations. For example, until released, criminals cannot vote or travel, the mentally incompetent cannot manage their affairs and those who are unlikely to ever achieve or re-achieve unambiguous self-consciousness may be allowed to die through compassionate withdrawal of food and medical treatment. Ultimately, one's competence as a human can be so diminished that one's rights as a human all but disappear. Conversely, were an individual animal to demonstrate the ability to discharge societal obligations expected of humans, such an animal could well make a logical claim for constitutional personhood in the United States (Rivard, p.1495).

Ultimately, Singer's thesis is valuable in raising awareness with regard to the need to *at least consider*, in any utilitarian balancing of interests, the pain and suffering of all sentient animals, especially those with possible self-consciousness. He falls short, however, by demanding that such a balancing accord *equal* consideration to entities with unambiguous capability for pain and suffering, such as humans, with entities that may or may not suffer in anything like the same way (rats?), and with some that almost certainly don't suffer at all but simply reflexively react to pain stimulus (worms?). Singer's theory can be rendered consistent with xenotransplantation by admitting into its utilitarian calculus the fact that humans *are known to* suffer more from disease than animals. This must be the case because we know human minds more than we know any animal mind, and because we are most certain of human self-awareness, and, consequently fear of impending death and disability. Even Singer admits, "A human dying from cancer is likely to suffer more than a mouse" (Singer, *Practical*, p.53).

Nuanced in this fashion, Singer's animal-inclusive utilitarianism raises no bar to pain-free explantation of xenografts from specially-bred and well-treated pigs. The good to humans of avoiding the death, disability, pain and suffering of end-stage organ failure more than outweighs the harm to an equal number of pigs of a painless death after a decent life. In each case a being dies, but pain and suffering has been avoided, so the total amount of "good" has been increased. In the same way, it can be argued that the good to pigs can also be increased due to the better conditions of breeding that should be associated with their use for medical purposes.

Regan: Don't Play the Weighing Game with Life

Many commentators disagree with the utilitarian balancing of interests. Disenchantment arises especially from the inability of utilitarianism to adequately protect minorities, and from the problematic nature of balancing interests in the face of incomplete information regarding what harms or benefits are actually in play. Tom Regan's classic *The Case for Animal Rights* attempts to derive an ideal philosophy from first principles. He settles on a deontological (i.e., the rules don't depend on the consequence of their application) theory of rights as his choice for an optimally parsimonious theory that systematizes human intuition as to right and wrong.

Regan's theory of rights proscribes the use of a sentient being as a means to an end. This theory is based on the concept that anything that is the "subject-of-a-life" has "inherent value." This inherent value gives rise to a right not to be harmed, including a right to protection from being harmed:

> [I]ndividuals are subjects-of-a-life if they have beliefs and desires; perceptions, memory, and a sense of the future, including their own future; an emotional life together with feelings of pleasure and pain; preference- and welfare-interests; the ability to initiate action in pursuit of their desires and goals; a psychophysical identity over time; and an individual welfare in the sense that their experiential life fares well or ill for them, logically independently of their utility for others and logically independently of their being the object of anyone else's interests (Regan, p.243).

Regan insists that all animals with self-awareness are "subjects-of-a-life" (and hence have inherent value), and that an unknown number of animals lacking self-awareness may also have inherent value. This expansiveness and vagueness creates serious problems of internal consistency and practicality. Inconsistency appears because while Regan clearly recognizes varying degrees of sentience, he adamantly refuses to recognize any associated differences in the quanta of respect for life that such differences entail:

> All animals [both human and non-human] are equal, when the notions of "animal" and "equality" are properly understood, "animal" referring to all (terrestrial, at least) moral agents and patients [again, human and non-human], and "equality" referring to their equal possession of inherent value. Inherent value is thus a categorical concept. One either has it, or one does not. There are no in-betweens. Moreover, all those who have it, have it equally. It does not come in degrees . . . . Injustice arises when we treat those who have such value in ways that fail to display proper respect (for example, by treating them as if their value was reducible to their utility for others) (Regan, pp.240-41, 264).

Regan fails to appreciate that it is possible – indeed, inevitable – for the lives of members of one species to be sacrificed for the benefit of members of other species. Midgely aptly identifies the errors of a Regan-type philosophy:

> Conflicts of interest must be recognized both within the human species and outside it. We have to take sides, and are entitled to put our own species first. All species do this. No creature can in fact subsist without killing some others, if only by competing with them for food. The point is not that we can hope to avoid injuring either animals or people. It is that we ought to recognize that such an injury matters, and to try to avoid it where no adequate reason justifies it (Midgely, p.223).

For example, if the needs of more sentient species affect other "subjects-of-a-life," as they inevitably will in a closed ecosystem, Regan offers no accommodation. He would have humans protect fish from bears. By according most every life form an equal quanta of "inherent value," without regard to whether impingements matter to them (such as the comatose patient, or perhaps the painlessly killed, well-bred, unaware animal), Regan provides society with no guidance as to the accommodation of conflicting interests among life forms. He also fails, thereby, to provide in practice a mechanism for respecting the "inherent value" of lives that he extols in theory.

Notwithstanding these weaknesses in Regan's theory, Regan does cast a good spotlight on a common concept needed for managing animal and human interests in xenotransplantation that all life has "inherent value" and hence should be respected. Regan takes this notion to an impractical end when he insists that "inherent value" is absolutely unimpingible. A better formulation of his deontological principle of inherent value would be that sentient lives may never *only* be a means to an end but must *also* be respected as ends in themselves, and this is so irrespective of the type of sentient animal we are referring to. In the xenotransplantation context this means that it is ethically appropriate to use pig organs to keep men alive, but only if the donor pig is provided with a meaningful life, and a respectful death, as well.

Generally, then, Regan's emphasis on the "inherent value" of animal life is useful to the degree that it reminds us of the necessity clearly to formulate the extent of our obligations toward each species, in a way based on characteristics most associated with the well-being of its members. What he does not demonstrate is the moral equality of all species in relation to the appropriateness of some members using other members to further their own critical interests. To benefit from Regan's contribution, while still clarifying the need to circumscribe the value of a being, this book uses the term "intrinsic value" instead of "inherent value" to refer to the morally special but conditionally sacrificial nature of all animal life.

Frey: Humans Outweigh Animals by a Longshot

Unlike both Regan and Singer, Raymond Frey takes head-on the manifold differences in quality of life among animals and men – and generally finds humans to have the much more valuable lives (Frey, *Rights*, p.108). Frey does not believe the term "animal rights" has meaning for ethical analysis (as the term "rights" is conventionally understood), and he also finds philosophical and logical problems with the phrase "animal interests." Frey subscribes to the utilitarian paradigm as does Singer, but comes to very different conclusions because of a much diminished moral worth accorded to non-human animals.

According to Frey, for an animal to have an interest it must have an ability to pursue that interest, or at least a potential ability to understand the interest (Frey, *Interests*, p.128). If it knows nothing of the interest, then it is no differently situated than, say an ancient tree that should not be cut down or a medieval rock formation that should not be defaced. We do not say that the tree or rock formations have "interests." Instead, it is human society that has an interest in preserving ancient trees and rock formations.

Frey's views are challengeable on the basis that humans also have interests of which they may be unaware. For example, a person's lack of awareness of detailed anti-pollution regulations, does not vitiate their interest in those regulations – especially if they help prevent cancer. And while Frey might counter that the person nevertheless has a potential ability to understand the interest, this argument does not apply to other persons (e.g. demented geriatric patients) who are definitely without this ability but to whom we continue to ascribe a wide range of interests that are the object of medical treatment. For another medical example, it is surely coherent to say that Type I diabetics in medieval Europe had an interest in the effective treatment of their condition (i.e. insulin) without being aware – or capable of being aware – of what that medicine may be. However, as Harris teaches, harming interests that an entity is unaware of must be weighed against concomitant harms to interests as to which an entity is aware (Harris, *Clones*, p.123). In the latter case, "double damage" is inflicted because both the interests are impugned as well as is the entity who is cognizant of those interests (Harris, *Clones*, p.123).

Frey observes that with regard to animals, it is human society that has the interests in how animals are treated. However, the presence of a human interest does not preclude the possibility of an animal interest. Animals demonstrate some of their interests by attempting to escape from painful situations. This does not mean, however, that animal interests are equivalent to human interests. The animal has an interest in life *per se*, simply by virtue of the instinct for survival, whether or not the animal is aware of it. However, this interest can be trumped by the human interest in survival because, as noted by Frey, self-conscious interests are the most important interests. In a similar vein, Harris denounces gratuitous harm to animals, but recognizes the moral legitimacy of harming their interests in life if "absolutely and unequivocally necessary in order to save a person's life or to prevent serious injury or suffering to persons" (Harris, *The Value*, pp.218-19).

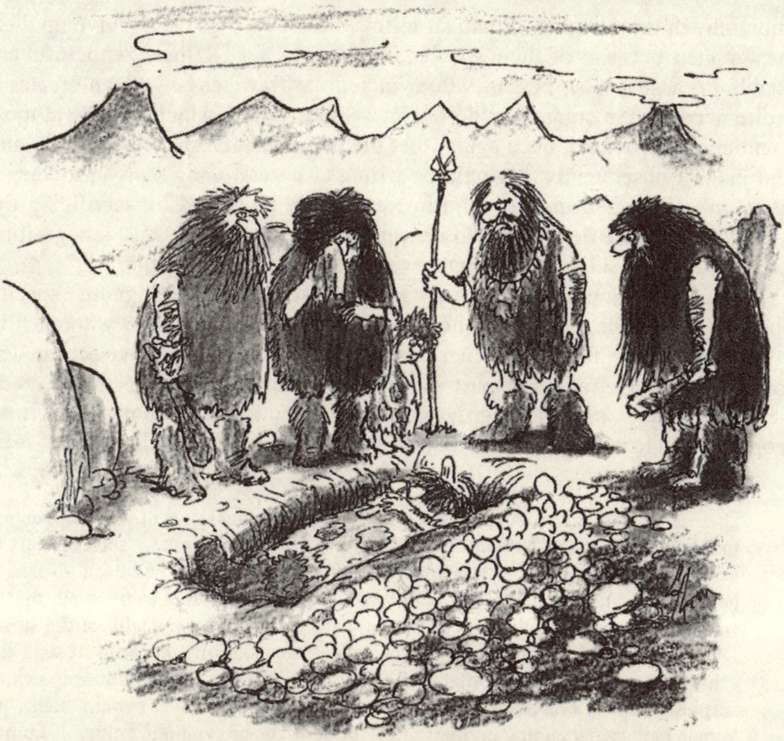

"We are comforted by the knowledge that at twenty-six years of age, he had lived a long and full life."

Like Singer, however, Frey believes that the utilitarian balancing of interests should include all interests – although he gives short shrift to concerns of animal welfare *per se* (because he believes animals lack interests *per se*) and is much more concerned with balancing competing human interests with regard to animal welfare. Hence Frey is of course willing to sacrifice animal lives for human lives since the former are presumptively much less valuable in an "enjoyment of life" sense than the latter. But he would also be willing to sacrifice human lives for animal (or other human lives) if the sacrificed human life is less valuable – due, for example, to a debilitating physical or mental infirmity – than the life to be saved (Frey, p.196). Frey's willingness to ignore species membership in ethical decision-making also poses no bar to xenotransplantation. The quality of a pig's life is vastly inferior to the quality of a typical human's life, and hence there is no bar to farming the pig's organs for the man. On the other hand, Frey would object to using a pig's organ to keep alive a comatose human, because the vegetative person has no quality of life (Frey, *Interests*, p.109).

Frey's thesis is consistent with recognizing the "intrinsic value" of all life as common ground between animal liberationists and human speciesists, pursuant to a hierarchy of moral value. Pursuant to this hierarchy, pigs do not give up their organs for men because of their species identity *per se*. Rather, xenografts are acceptable because *known* human values include self-awareness, which creates a more dire need for the organ than do the known pig values, which include at most only sentience – provided, once again, that the organ is harvested respectfully and without pain. Consequently, it would be wrong to harvest a pig's organ to keep a comatose man alive because no valid interest would be served by sacrificing the pig. And, if pigs were determined to be as self-aware as are humans, xenografting their organs even for self-aware humans would cease to be acceptable.

The unwillingness of Frey, Regan and Singer to ignore species membership is troubling to those who see an invitation to barbarism without firm lines drawn between man and other animals. Observing that vivisection was outlawed in Nazi Germany as part of an "Aryan oneness with Nature" credo (including anti-smoking campaigns, bans on alcohol, glorification of German homeopathy, and iconification of certain animals), Deborah Rudacille writes:

> Does an elevation in the moral status of animals inevitably result in a degradation in the moral status of human beings? Certainly in Nazi Germany such appears to be the case. Once the distinction between human and animal had been leveled, it became possible to conceive of breeding humans in the same way that a conscientious farmer might breed his animals, to improve the health of the stock. Diseased or weak or otherwise unwanted humans could be disposed of with the same lack of moral feeling that one might experience in "putting down" sick or surplus beasts. Certain species of animals could be valued over certain "races" of human beings, depending on their utility or aesthetic or symbolic value. If human life and animal life were morally equivalent, acts that had previously been unthinkable could become commonplace (Rudacille, pp.89-90).

The problem with the quoted passage is that it leaps from "elevating the moral status of animals" to "moral equivalency" of the species. The importance of the intrinsic value concept is that it emphasizes treating all animals with respect, and yet permits discrimination in favor of humans because indisputable self-consciousness demands yet *more* respect. The moral gap between people and animals still remains huge even after elevating animals to a moral status that precludes the imposition of unnecessary pain (Harris, *The Value*, p.219). Humans enjoy many more benefits than merely the avoidance of being caused pain by someone else. Respect describes a broad continuum of behaviors, and it need not be completely withheld from animals, or too parsimoniously allocated, in order to remain a highly valuable good.

There still remains the issue of how do we *know* that only humans experience self-consciousness, and are thus entitled to special moral treatment? One school of thought teaches that the answer lies in the uniquely human ability of language.

Leahy: Weigh it in Words

Unlike Frey, Regan opted out of comparing human and animal lives because he viewed all subjects-of-a-life to have equal inherent value. Some linguistic philosophers, such as Michael Leahy, also opt out of comparing human and animal lives – their reason, however, is that animals without language lead such meaningless lives that it would be irrational to compare them in any way to human lives. Does animals' lack of language ability preclude any kind of self-consciousness? If so, does this mean that they can be mere instrumentalities with no welfare interests of their own?

Leahy develops a trenchant case that one cannot conceptualize even "suffering" or other facets of self-consciousness without the tools of syntax and vocabulary. In essence, Leahy recapitulates Descartes' "I think therefore I am" as "I have language, therefore I am":

> Clearly animals, unlike plants, are conscious; but self-consciousness, like hope, ambition, remorse, and envy, come only with the capability of speech (Leahy, p.166).

There are two reasons to bow to Leahy's logic. First, it *is* difficult to imagine what would go on in the mind of an entity that had no symbol system with which to label, arrange and rearrange reality. Here is how George Orwell endeavored to explain a gunshot wound, in images that might be as appropriate for a deer as to a man:

> Roughly speaking it was the sensation of being at the center of an explosion. There seemed to be a loud bang and a blinding flash of light all around me, and I felt a tremendous shock – no pain, only a violent shock, such as you get from an electric terminal; with it a sense of utter weakness, a feeling of being stricken and shriveled up to nothing (Orwell, p.177).

But if we are reacting to Orwell's words, then we are already one step removed from a deer that can only feel the sensation. Is the sensation the same without words to name it? Certainly when we hurt ourselves, the sensation does not have to first be expressed in a lexicon to hurt. Nevertheless, Leahy insists that if nothing is named, the relationship of self to the external world is unabstractable, and Descartes was correct in saying that all that remained was biological programming (Leahy, p.166). The resemblance of animal programmed reflexes to human reflexes no more gives rise to self-consciousness than does an artist's self portrait (or portrait of another) have the artist's (or anyone's) *actual* personality. The painting may invoke *in our minds* a personality, but of course the canvas is not alive. Similarly, the animal sound may invoke *in our minds* a "wimper," but, to linguistic philosophers such as Leahy, the dog can't "feel sad" without a lexicon and syntax.

How Much Does Private Language Count?

A counter-argument may be raised here based on the concept of "private language." Wittgenstein coined the notion that "sounds which no one else understands but which I *'appear to understand'* might be called a private language" (Wittgenstein, p.94). Hence, it could be said that just because animals don't speak anything that we believe to be a language, it does not follow that they do not have a language and a vocabulary to support pain. Similarly, it could be imagined that some people have words for concepts or sensations that they, and nobody else, understands: Even if every person had a different meaning for the word pain, in order to communicate about pain, they would still have to agree on a publicly accessible definition for pain, such as that sensation that causes writhing, howling, or certain types of crying. Whatever the private definition of pain, to Wittgenstein, it does not constitute language. Instead, private definitions, like private language in general, are terms that apply to vague personal feelings but not to words and meanings. Words, in the Wittgenstein conceptualization, achieve meaning only through social intercourse. The concept of a purely private language is, in fact, illusory.

Physiological Signs of Pain

The absence of a private language "name" for animal pain does not imply that our perception of animal pain is fictitious. To the contrary, Wittgenstein is adamant that the concept of "pain" is intimately connected to publicly accessible language that, in turn, is intimately connected with human society. "Language, in Wittgenstein's later view, does not merely reflect reality; in significant measure it constitutes the world" (Rubinstein, p.170). Neither the private language argument, nor its demolition by Wittgenstein, resolves the issue of whether animals suffer. However, Wittgenstein does make clear that physical acts, previously associated with words, can serve as symbols of the meanings attached to those words. When we see the animal writhe like a human being writhes when in pain, we interpret that *publicly accessible* sign of pain as what we have repeatedly had confirmed in our lives to mean "pain."

Consequently, if one does not believe an animal is writhing as a game, then one reasonably concludes – subject to cross-species uncertainty and ambiguity – that the writhing reflects a sensation similar to what we call pain. This is because everyone has grown up to associate writhing behavior with pain, notwithstanding any other linguistic references or semantic capabilities. In a similar vein, we do not doubt that a stroke patient *can* suffer severe pain despite the possibility that all semantic conceptualizations of pain were erased from his mind by the stroke. But we only *believe* that the stroke patient *is* suffering pain when the *doctor persuades us that the patient must be suffering pain* because of certain anatomical or neurological reasons. The doctor's expertise functions like the animal's writhing – it is a publicly accessible communication that we understand.

It may be the case that animals *perceive* what humans call pain differently than humans because of our different communication abilities or, more generally, neurological wiring. For the animals, sensations similar to what we call pain may have the texture that can be encapsulated in a howl, whimper or writhe. For the humans, pain may have all of those textures, as well as those enabled by the rich lexicon of publicly accessible words. But the same kind of neurons that transfer pain signals to the brain in humans exist in our evolutionary mammalian cousins. *Consequently, the physiological basis for what we verbalize as pain, exists, at least in amputated form, in animals as well.* Leahy's language-defines-pain argument is therefore useful but only when transcended to underline our ability to use language to recognize pain in animals and to accord related levels of respect to all animal life.

Only Language Separates Us From Them

The second language lesson Leahy brings to bear on animal "liberationist" doctrine relates to line-drawing. If language is not the dividing line between sentience and automata, then where does one stop in separating beings with interests from inanimate (or at least disregardable) things? Why respect chimps but not pigs, pigs but not rats, rats but not worms, worms but not bacteria? All of these react to undesired stimuli evasively, although none demonstrate any ability abstractly to conceptualize their experience. If language is not the dividing line for beings with interests, Leahy argues, then life would be absurd. For we practically cannot and do not accord respect to worms or bacteria. We exterminate rats; we eat pigs, and we cage chimps.

The liberationists are undaunted by what they consider to be linguistic legerdemain (one is reminded of Wittgenstein's warning that "Philosophy is a battle against the bewitchment of our intelligence by means of language" (Wittgenstein, part. 109)). The issue, they claim, is not whether animals have language skills. The issue is whether animals are entitled to protection from human domination for human benefit because the animals are living creatures with, in various people's views, capacity for suffering, emotion, or self-consciousness. They refuse to concede that language is the portal to self-consciousness, suffering, intrinsic value or protectable interests. The liberationists either analogize animals to mentally deficient humans, or simply assert as a given that animals have an "inherent value" that constitutes a protectable interest.

There is also a further critique of Leahy, Wittgenstein and others of the "I speak therefore I am" school. This critique shares some of the liberationist concerns about animal welfare (though by no means all) and identifies a major flaw in the logic that says it is language ability, *per se*, that separates man from all else – *res cogitans* from *res extensa*. The flaw is failing to recognize that language and thought must arise from experience, and that the animal kingdom is a vital part of human experience.

> Nothing can be understood on its own. Had we known no other animate life-form than our own, we should have been utterly mysterious to ourselves as a species. And that would have made it immensely harder for us to understand ourselves as individuals too. Anything that puts us in context, that shows us as part of a continuum, an example of a type that varies on intelligible principles, is a great help. People welcome seeing how animals behave, either directly or on film, in just the same way in which a man who had begun to practice, say, mathematics or dancing on his own would welcome seeing others who were already doing it, though differently (Midgely, p.18).

In other words, the very language-thought complex, which Leahy and others rely upon as the talisman of human uniqueness, is, in fact, totally infected with animal world experience. Hence, when we hurt animals, we also hurt ourselves in some way. A strict Cartesian separation of species is illusory. This fact is yet further driven home when one considers the collective, social nature of even a single human mind:

> [T]he mind has a collective existence – a shared ideal of individuality towards which particular persons aspire, in order to define themselves for themselves and for others . . . . Without the mirror that the actions and utterances of others supply, it is inconceivable that you could ever grasp what manner of thing you yourself might be or become . . . . Thus the philosophically abstract conception of the self-sufficiency of the individual mind, free and independent of others, serves to conceal its origins as a social product of rule-governed reflection. "I think therefore I am" totally obscures the social process whereby the use of the term "I" is acquired (Doyal and Harris, p.86).

This interactionist model of human development shows that if language uniquely gives humans the capacity to feel pain and suffering, it is only because that language has become infused with personal meaning via interaction with a social environment in which non-human animals constitute a primary reference grid. Consequently, when humans cause pain to animals they are causing pain to a human-animal psycho-social relationship that ultimately finds expression in the mind of every person (Kant, p.241). It is the failure to take common human-animal "mindspace" into account that saps Leahy's thesis of its real world relevance. Indeed, insisting that humans are not part of a broader ecosystem is bound to impoverish any theory:

> The really monstrous thing about Existentialism too is its proceeding as if the world contained only dead matter (things) on the one hand and fully rational, educated, adult human beings on the other – as if there were no other life-forms. The impression of desertion or abandonment which Existentialists have is due, I am sure, not to the removal of God, but to this contemptuous dismissal of almost the whole biosphere – plants, animals, and children. Life shrinks to a few urban rooms; no wonder it becomes absurd (Midgely, p.19).

Giving Darwin Some Respect

We thus arrive at a canyon of chasms – one school of scholars would not deem animals to be self-conscious and capable of suffering (in the human sense of the term) even erring on the side of caution. To this school of thought, the undeniable lack of language skills among pigs is conclusive evidence that they are mere automata. A second school of scholars deems animals to be self-conscious and capable of human-type suffering without even approaching the gray zone of caution. To this group, animal squealing, writhing and escape when harm is caused to them is conclusive evidence that they are not automata:

> no truth appears to me more evident, than that the beasts are endow'd with thought and reason as well as man. The arguments are in this case so obvious, that they never escape the most stupid and ignorant (Hume, I.176).

Yet a third group urges recognition of an animal-human continuum that ricochets harm to animals back into man via the socially collective nature of self-consciousness. The pro-animal rights school denies that they are being tricked by "language games" into interpreting "humanish" animal reflexes as human feelings. And as to line drawing, they either take an absolutist position and avoid harm to any kind of animal life except in self-defense (antibiotics are acceptable if one is being attacked by bacteria), or they "err on the side of caution" and condone wanton harm to worms, but not to rats, because the latter evidence more convincing signs of pain than do the former.

Notwithstanding the hard line drawn by "languagists", there is common ground to be found. Even the most radical debunkers of animal liberation, those who believe that language forms a Rubicon between self-consciousness and automata, concede out of respect for Darwin that higher animal life are "primitive beings" that "exhibit the pre-linguistic sensations of pain and the ancestral tokens of human attributes such as deliberative intent, rational planning, choice, desire, fear, anger, and some beliefs, where our guiding criteria are the close similarity of their behavioural patterns, in like circumstances, to our own" (Leahy, p.166). Since a mature "languaged" being has non-instrumental value, it would seem difficult to deny that a primitive being had some of this value as well, albeit of a lesser quality, quantity or kind. Indeed, because animals are undeniably an evolutionary stump of humans, a strong argument exists that they also share a stump of human moral worth. A corollary to Leahy's begrudged grant of "primitive being" status to animals is at least a partial grant of non-instrumental value to their lives. Leahy's "primitive being" conceptualization paves the way for a recognition that language skills are not the *sine qua non* to be valued as more than merely a means to an end.

Ronald Dworkin provides a theoretical bridge across the animal rights chasms with his concept of the "intrinsic value" of life – an isoform of the term adopted by Tom Regan in his deontological theory of absolute non-interference with all sentient life forms. Writing in the context of the abortion debate, Dworkin teaches that the real issue is not whether a fetus is a patient, but rather how do we interpret in our own life the "intrinsic value" of the fetus as incipient life (Dworkin 1994, pp.23, 67). Dworkin's conceptualization is readily transferable to the animal welfare issue in xenotransplantation. *The key moral question is how should we accommodate our intuitive feelings that all higher animal life has intrinsic value*?

We must accept in a secular society that there will be different interpretations of when an intrinsic value can be sacrificed for personal needs. It is reasonable for a society built upon common cultural sentiments to draw some outer boundaries of what interpretations are acceptable. But it is equally important in a secular society to leave a broad range of decision-making about an essentially religious concept up to the internal moral compasses of individuals. "The realm of what a free society should permit is not coextensive with the realm of what a free society should approve on moral grounds" (Harris, "The Ethics," p.323). In this way, society can proscribe late-term abortions, and proscribe interference with early-term abortions, while still countenancing religious and cultural teaching about the intrinsic value of fetal life.

Applied to animal welfare, Dworkin would have us realize that, in a secular society, different people must be permitted to have different interpretations of the essentially religious notion that animal life has intrinsic value (Dworkin 1994, p.67). It is reasonable for our society to draw some outer boundaries as a matter of law – such as the avoidance of cruelty to pig organ donors, and the avoidance of interference with xenotransplantation programs. But it is also important for people to realize that the disagreements over degrees of acceptable impingement upon an animal's intrinsic value are "at bottom spiritual," and "that real community is possible across deep religious divisions" (Dworkin 1994, p.101).[1] A Dworkin-inspired paradigm of moral value could be charted as follows:

Principle: All sentient beings have intrinsic value.

Principle: Avoid suffering of sentient beings.

Corollary: Avoid unwanted death of self-conscious subset of sentient beings since such deaths entail suffering.

Corollary: It is morally acceptable to kill non-self-conscious beings without causing them suffering in order to alleviate suffering in a self-conscious being (i.e. xenotransplantation).

---

[1] Interestingly, the major religions that forbid eating pork have all come out in favor of xenotransplantation using pig organs (Vanderpool 2001, p.141).

> *Questions for scientific research and/or religious belief*: Which animals are self-conscious, and to what degree? What constitutes suffering beyond frank pain?

Advocates of xenotransplantation must concede that they are treading on sacred ground in using animal organs. Too many people accord animals intrinsic value to argue otherwise. Consequently, the animals should be treated with respect. On the other hand, advocates of animal rights must concede that we do not live in a liberationist theocracy. There is little ideological consistency to the intrinsic value interpretations that people vest in animals. Consequently, individual use of a xenograft, like individual consumption of meat, is a question best addressed by the conscience of an individual, not the dictate of a State. However, because of the consensus that the human interest in xenotransplantation trumps the intrinsic value which we also attribute to a pig's life, the establishment and regulation of xenotransplantation should be a matter for the State and not the individual.

Chimerism and Its Discontents

In the following section it will be shown that the treatment of pigs in practice follows the Dworkin conceptualization quite well: the intrinsic value of pigs is protected at the boundary by government regulations, but within those limits there is a great amount of freedom for individual conscience. There is a balance between recognizing the intrinsic value of animals (e.g., frank cruelty proscribed) and recognizing the fundamentally religious nature of how to interpret that value (e.g., vegetarianism is a personal, often spiritual, decision). Many fewer pigs will be raised and killed for xenotransplantation. Here, too, there will be a balance between respecting the intrinsic value of pigs (e.g., treat transgenic pigs with "kid gloves"), and not forcing on anyone a particular, essentially religious, interpretation of that value (e.g., no one will be forced to use xenografts).

Nevertheless, the hybridization of porcine and human biosystems for xenotransplantation is certain to give rise to discontent. If someone feels, as a matter of principle, that combining two species is wrong, then they will not be pleased with any humanization of the pig genome, or with millions of pigs' hearts beating in human chests. This chapter also seeks to clarify that hybridization without "monstrous" results is part and parcel of nature, and thus nothing to fear or loathe. There is no prospect that xenotransplantation would proceed in the wake of "monstrous" results, such as talking pigs or squealing men.

Piled High and Deep: The Realities of Pork

In the United Kingdom, approximately 3 million animals are used annually in research laboratories, down from around 5 million employed annually in the 1970s. In the US, comparable figures are 100 million annually in the early 1980s and 90 million annually in the early 1990s (Rudacille, p.124). Rats and mice account for 75-80 percent; dogs and cats together are less than 1 percent, and the balance are smaller rodents, fish and birds, and an extremely small number of larger mammals.

The use of animals for food dwarfs all other uses. In the UK, approximately 400 million animals are killed for food each year. Of pigs in particular, 7.6 million were slaughtered for food in the US in the single month of November 1996, implying nearly 100 million pigs per year are consumed in or exported from the US for food (Cooper and Lanza, p.50). Consequently, whatever interests liberationist theorists believe pigs to have, society does not recognize such interests or rights to the extent of protecting pigs from being eaten. It would seem, therefore, that animal rights advocates would be hard-pressed to prevent a vastly fewer number of pigs from being sacrificed just by a ban on xenografts. Were all deaths in the U.S. due to heart failure prevented with a xenograft, approximately one million pigs annually would be sacrificed for a medical reason – about 1 percent of the number slaughtered for food.

Unlimited eating of animals, ironically, is not viewed by society as inconsistent with the adoption of detailed rules for the "humane treatment" of laboratory animals. Animal rights groups have succeeded in getting legislation and regulations adopted that sharply circumscribe the nature of experimental procedures that can be conducted on animals (7 U.S.C. §2143 (1999) (Federal Animal Welfare Act).

Notwithstanding the success of animal rights groups in pushing anti-cruelty laws through the legislative process, they stand very little chance of passing similar laws to block xenotransplantation based on the rights or interests of pigs. This conclusion is based on the historical record. For nearly two hundred years anti-vivisectionists and their allies have agitated on behalf of animal rights, but all that the public ever accepts are laws that prohibit cruelty toward animals, not their killing. Similarly, in the United States, agitation by animal rights groups has resulted in heightened criminal penalties for animal cruelty. The crime is now a felony in 27 states, with fines up to $100,000 and prison terms up to ten years, whereas only six years ago animal cruelty was a minor misdemeanor in most states (Glaberson, p.1). However, the anti-cruelty laws "typically declare that people cannot be prosecuted for standard farming practices, like beef slaughtering" (Glaberson, p.16). In a similar vein, amendments passed in 1985 to the U.S. Federal Animal Welfare Act said conditions of confinement must assure "the psychological well being of primates" (Glaberson, p.16). Note that the obligation is toward avoiding cruelty (isolation in this case), not toward vesting the animal with a right of freedom. Consequently, it can be reasonably expected that the practical thrust of the animal rights movement will be to ensure that xenograft donor pigs are treated "humanely" before being sacrificed. This is a high likelihood in any event given the need to ensure the animals are raised in SPF conditions and the fact that the animals are far more valuable than hogs destined to become food.

Pigs raised under conditions of "intensive farming" (highly crowded, assembly-line meat production) are known to gnaw at the hide of other pigs in their crowded pen. The advent of the animal rights movement has had little effect on the popularity of intensive farming, which of course must be accomplished in full accordance with national law. By comparison, xenograft pigs will be raised in facilities that are subject to inspection and approval by Government regulators of biopharmaceutical products. Given the concern with having disease-free pigs as organ donors, and in light of the asceptic conditions that prevail for biopharmaceutical products generally, it is logical to assume that xenograft herds would readily meet any conditions that animal rights agitators succeeded in getting adopted for the pork industry.

In summary, animal rights advocates have achieved great progress in some countries in ensuring that animals are not treated cruelly, at least compared to historical standards or to sadistic-type behavior. This accomplishment reflects the growing recognition in such countries that animals, including pigs, have "intrinsic value." However, liberationists have made no legislative progress in persuading countries that it is inappropriate to treat pigs as primarily a means to satisfy human needs for food, research, or medicine. Provided that these ends can be achieved without cruelty, it appears as if the public is willing to accept it.

Transgressing the Pig Genome

Aside from animal welfare objections, it is also possible that a constituency could gather around opposition to the chimerism that is inherent in xenotransplantation. Chimerism means the hybridization of two or more species. Since such hybridization cannot occur through natural procreative means, it is often criticized as being "unnatural" and, depending on how strange the results appear, abhorrent. There are several levels of chimerism to consider: (1) humanizing the pig's DNA to avoid hyperacute rejection; (2) introducing porcine biochemistry into a human organ recipient via the pig organ and (3) the psychological realization that one has a pig organ.

To the extent that xenografts violate the "natural order of life," there is opposition to the technology on quasi-religious grounds that chimerism is, *per se*, morally wrong. However, a closer examination of each aspect of chimerism will reveal it to be a morally neutral activity. In addition, as the "tree of life" figure indicates below, all life is fundamentally chimeric. The intermixing of all life arises from the evolutionary process by which every species, genus, family, order, class, phylum and kingdom branches from, and hence partially incorporates, another. Anti-chimeric sentiment is fundamentally a position that opposes any *additional* admixture of species beyond that which has "naturally" evolved. Depending on the advocate, chimerism might be wrong for animals but acceptable in plants, wrong in primates but acceptable in domesticated beasts, or perhaps just wrong if the human species is involved.

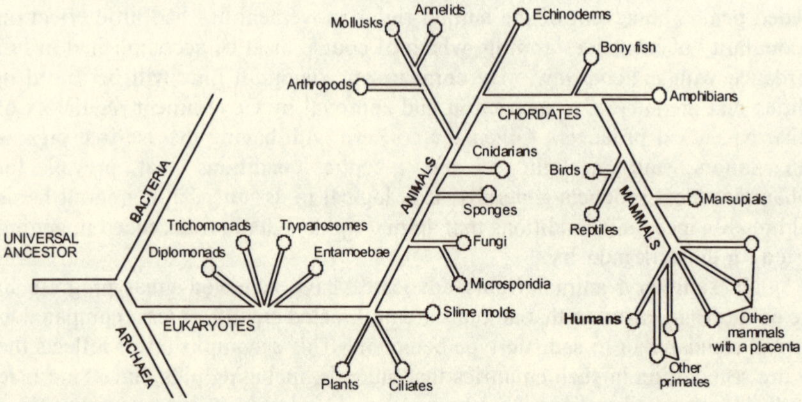

Figure IV-1 Evolutionary Tree

First, donor pigs' organs must be genetically modified via transgenic engineering in order to avoid hyperacute rejection by the human immune system. In essence, scientists slightly humanize the pig's organs at the level of the pig's germ cell DNA. This enables an entire herd of transgenic pigs to be created, each of which will have organs that avoid hyperacute rejection when transplanted into humans. The general procedure is to splice certain human genes, which code for immune system proteins, onto the pig genome, and/or to delete from the pig genome certain pig genes that code for proteins especially noxious to the human immune system. The issues are whether this bit of genetic engineering has (1) harmed the pigs, or (2) violated the "natural order of things" in some immoral way.

Pigs born with transgenic DNA are not expected to be different in any way from non-transgenic pigs, except with regard to a few immune system proteins. The public has not accepted the view that individual pigs have any rights or interests except to be spared cruelty. Since the transgenic modification causes no pig reaction that is even interpretable as pain, or shortens the pig's lifespan, it is safely concluded that the genetic engineering has not, in any tangible sense, harmed the pig.

It could be posited that the pig species has been harmed by an unrequested and unnatural genetic transposition. However, this objection fails to recognize that all pigs are not being modified – the modification occurs only in the very small percentage of pigs that are destined to be used as organ donors. In addition, humans have long modified pig DNA via selective breeding. It is therefore most unlikely that a public consensus would gather around the notion that transgenics harms the pig species, since the entire species is not being modified. Instead, a new sub-species, effectively a breed, is being created. There is a romanticized notion that selective breeding is "natural" and that transgenics is not. But such a romanticized notion must take into account that pigs do not live "natural" lives in free range environments. If the public were to rise up and oppose xenotransplantation based on "unnatural" modifications being affected on the pig species, they would also have to rise up to protest the "unnatural" lives virtually all pigs lead in "unnatural" environments.

As noted earlier in discussing Dworkin, what may appear as speciesism in xenotransplantation is, instead, simply an implementation of respect for the intrinsic value of all life. The unambiguously self-conscious human is spared the suffering of end-stage organ failure. The pig's experience, though different depending upon the view taken, is also painless. From one perspective, the probably not self-conscious, but quite sentient, pig is spared suffering during its life and is oblivious to the time and manner of death. An alternative perspective is that the pig does not experience suffering in the first place, so the modifications would never be incorporated into its consciousness.

Finally, an important difference needs to be highlighted between genetically modified (GM) food and xenografts. Public opposition to GM food rests on the facts that it is ingested (1) by all; (2) involuntarily in many if not most cases and (3) unnecessarily since most ate well with non-GM techniques. A correlative objection to GM seeds for insect resistance is that they were implemented with "terminator" characteristics that fundamentally changed the economics of farming – the occupation of the majority of people in developing countries. None of these facts apply to genetically modified pig organs. They will be used only by the infirm, only in conjunction with informed consent, and only if there is no other way to save the person's life. There is little reason to expect the public's opposition to GM foods to spillover into prohibitions against genetically modified pig organs. However, the term "genetic modification" undoubtedly will retain a negative aura for many, and it is this negative connotation that may be picked up by opinion polls.

Transgressing Humanity

The second facet of chimerism introduced by xenotransplantation is the introduction of porcine biochemistry into humans. The basic concern is that, once again, but with higher stakes, there is a violation of the "natural order of things" in mixing pig and human cells together. There is also a more far-fetched concern that some pig DNA would travel to the gonads of a human organ recipient, get integrated into that person's germ cell DNA, and, if the person had any offspring, that those offspring could be (even ever so slightly) human-pig chimeras.[2] One expert in the field casts the problem as follows:

---

[2] For a literary look at the possibilities of human-animal chimeras, see Mikhai Bulgahov's *Heart of a Dog*, a fantasy in which a human pituitary gland is implanted in a dog, who transforms into a model Russian citizen, except for a subconscious urge to kill cats.

> There are many issues that make people uncomfortable about xenotransplantation. At a very fundamental level it seems to transgress those boundaries which define us as human, and so challenge and threaten our identity and sense of order; the sense of order and disorder, according to some anthropologists, is the very basis of our entire cognitive world (Daar, p.77).

Others argue that the boundaries transgressed by xenografts are arbitrary constructions, fictions born of a pre-xeno technology:

> What is constituted as an individual within postmodern, biotechnical, biomedical discourse? There is no easy answer to this question, for even the most reliable Western individuated bodies, the mice and men of a well-equipped laboratory, neither stop nor start at the skin, which is itself something of a teeming jungle threatening illicit fusions, especially from the perspective of a scanning electron microscope (Haraway, p.215).

Haraway is saying that what we think of as a boundary is based, in part, on what we know from technology. However, she goes further and explains that technology is not the only arbiter of boundarylessness. For example, race and gender, once considered frozen based on "natural boundaries," are now constructed as:

> ideologies of human diversity . . . to be developed in terms of frequencies of parameters and fields of power-charged differences, not essences and natural origins or homes. Race and sex, like individuals, are artifacts sustained or undermined by the discursive nexus of knowledge and power. Any objects or persons can be reasonably thought of in terms of disassembly and reassembly; no "natural" architectures constrain system design . . . . No objects, spaces, or bodies are sacred in themselves; any component can be interfaced with any other if the proper standard, the proper code, can be constructed for processing signals in a common language . . . . In particular, there is no ground for ontologically opposing the organic, the technical, and the textual . . . . Bodies have become cyborgs – cybernetic organisms – compounds of hybrid techno-organic embodiment and textuality (Haraway, p.212).

The fact that Haraway drives home is the utter vacuosness of arguments against xenotransplantation that are based on "transgressing natural boundaries." To the degree that such boundaries do exist in nature, they may be ever more trangressed as technology succeeds in translating ever more biological codes. Consequently, the "natural boundaries" argument amounts to an ideological position that arbitrarily freezes in history the parameters of some boundaries that can be shown to be, to a degree, technologically fluid. Such ideologies may compete with others for prevalence in a society, but they cannot defensibly or objectively claim moral high ground. They also have scant chance of succeeding in a quest for an *apartheid*-like separation of animals from men in transplantation when the species merge in food, clothing, medicine, companionship and entertainment.

In retreat, defenders of the "natural boundaries" argument may complain that leather soles and household pets are not as intimate a boundary transgression as is a transplanted organ. But such an argument is no defense against human consumption of cooked and raw animal flesh that ultimately finds its way to every part of the body. And if finally it is urged that the human gastrointestinal tract sterilizes consumed animal kingdom invaders, there is the long list of diseases that show the porosity of these defenses. One might also add the mass vaccinations of human societies with fragments of animal virus DNA to beef up the human immune system:

> In the same way that the (pharmacologically suppressed) immune system gradually integrates a donated organ, there exists a cultural immune system which can be slowly modified. What initially is assessed as threatening is gradually integrated into the culture. An illustrative example is vaccination with cow-pox virus in the 17th century, which demonstrated that people's fear of developing animal characteristics, since the vaccine contained virus from cows, was steadily transformed into perceptions of a safe and self-evident treatment . . . . This interplay between cultural rejection and cultural integration also means that a new outlook on mankind can arise. It is tempting to formulate it like this: The biotechnological body is transformed to normality, while the natural defective body becomes abnormal (Lundin, pp.152-53).

The U.S. Congress analyzed the issue of how transgenics can blur human-animal boundaries, and concluded that practical boundaries would still be easily enough definable:

> The Committee recognizes the complexity of biotechnology and the possibility of placing human genes into nonhumans or nonhuman genes into humans. As in many scientific endeavors, the results may be difficult to predict. Yet, throughout history, humankind has been able to differentiate between human beings and nonhuman beings. And, of course, if a more precise definition is necessary in the future, the Congress then can discharge its responsibilities to craft new legislation (H.R. Rep., p.29).

Critics still worry that the "line dividing human and nonhuman will disappear; it will be replaced by a genetic continuum," and "the term 'human being' thus becomes inherently ambiguous" (Rivard, p.333). However, from the standpoint of our analysis into the feasibility of xenotransplantation addressing the organ gap, it doesn't much matter whether the boundary between humans and non-humans is becoming ambiguous, has always been ambiguous, or is "naturally" unambiguous. The important point is that because of people's overarching desire to remain alive, there appears to be only the slightest possibility of public opposition to xenotransplantation based on the transcending of species boundaries (Lundin, p.151). Anti-chimerism is either too esoteric or too incredible a concept around which a public consensus can congeal, especially as compared to the tangible life-saving benefits of xenografts.

Transgressive Psychology

One last non-scientific objection to xenotransplantation is that people may refuse the organs as undignified, or may suffer adverse psychological affects due simply to thinking about their porcine origin. The issue of potentially transgressive psychology seems more appropriate as an informed consent disclosure than as a non-scientific reason to impede xenotransplantation. It seems hardly credible that many would rather die than risk some ridicule or undergo psychological counseling as a consequence of a xenotransplant. For example, "due to the shared belief concerning the supreme value of preserving human life, Judaism, Catholicism, Protestantism, and Islam offer no principled objections to animal-to-human transplants" (Vanderpool 1999, p.155). Hence, a xenograft recipient can expect to receive family as well as community support for their decision, factors that will militate against any psychological misgivings. In addition, newly tightened xenograft clinical trial standards eschew premature experiments in which animal organs are placed into humans with virtually no chance of success ("Xenotransplantation Subcommittee"). These standards now specify that before human xenotransplantation can occur "the success rate of experimental pig-to-nonhuman primate transplants should be 90 percent survival for 2 months and 50 percent for 3 months" (Vanderpool 2001, p.141). A 2-3 month survival period will provide the patient with a good second chance at the allotransplant waiting list. Hopefully, the xenografts will function for ever longer periods of time and eventually moot the need for an allograft.

Even though the risk of transgressive psychology is unlikely to deter a person in need of a xenograft, there remains the issue of whether it could serve as an organizing theme for public opposition to xenotransplantation.

Given the closely controlled nature of clinical studies, it seems quite unlikely that any xenograft procedure that produced "frankenstein" personalities would get very far at all. Consequently, even if the public does get frightened by the "frankenstein factor" of modern medicine creating thousands of post-transplant porcine-minded citizens, that fright will in all likelihood be addressed by tighter scrutiny over limited clinical trials. Literature-induced fears that can readily be managed with normal public controls are unlikely to generate the public consensus needed to stop a beneficial medical procedure (Cassileth et al., p.148). Neither individual occurrences of transgressive psychology, nor the public's fear of it, will pull the plug on xenotransplantation.

Conclusion: No Revolution Likely on the Animal Pharm

This chapter has made clear that "animal rights" advocates and detractors arrive with radically different assumptions. Similarly, "natural order" supporters and debunkers do not accept the validity of each other's premises. Nevertheless, the apparent essential contestability of these paradigms can be bridged. Common ethical ground is found by recognizing that there is a shared belief that at least higher animal life has intrinsic value. Upon this common ground a paradigm-bridging structure consists of seeing disagreements over *how to respect the intrinsic value of life* as being *fundamentally religious* decisions. In a secular society it is expected, and even desired, that provisions be made for diverse religious beliefs. In the xenotransplantation context this means permissibility of xenografts on the one hand, but also lack of pain or suffering – or at least what we perceive to be pain or suffering – for the porcine organ donor on the other. Additionally, nobody should be required to choose a xenograft over the alternative of death or prolonged suffering.

Xenotransplantation has emerged relatively unscathed from the assessments of the past two chapters into disease-causing risks and non-scientific harms. Previously, xenografts had emerged as the best technical solution for solving the real organ gap. Now we know that xenogeneic disease risk is manageable, and that opposition constituencies can agree to respect individual decisions of conscience as to the use of xenografts, provided that society respects, at some basic level, the intrinsic value of at least higher animal life forms. So now the discussion may proceed to the ultimate question of whether humans have a right to xenotransplantation technology. If so, what should be done to respect that right?

Chapter V

The Right to Life: Society's Obligation to Provide Health Care and Xenotransplantation

Not all things are done that can be done. We have seen in chapters II through IV that xenotransplantation is feasible, with manageable risks and social tolerability. But it does not necessarily follow that the public *should* bow to the needs of a million or so deathly ill persons each year and provide them with a few more years of life. Thus, the issue to be addressed in this chapter is whether there is a right to xenotransplantation. Is there an obligation for the social provision of this procedure, and if so, how strict is it?

Introduction

There is a clear sense that people have some sort of entitlement to an organ transplant. Otherwise, so much concern would not exist over organ transplant waiting lists, and governments would not be so engaged in encouraging organ donation. This sense of entitlement must be based upon some sort of a *right* because rights discourse is a primary way to talk about entitlement. But what kind of right? And what corresponding duties are imposed on society to support that right?

There clearly is also a great *need* for many sick people to have an organ transplant. This need is of special importance because death is the usual result of its non-satisfaction. Addressing this special need therefore becomes an *issue of justice* because there are not enough organs to go around. The goal of this chapter is to unpack the issues of *rights, needs and justice* that intersect in the context of xenotransplantation.

Ought Implies Kant

Individual rights began to be recognized in the earliest human civilizations, but experienced a surge of growth in the 18th century – the limits of this expansion of freedom have yet to be seen. A trigger for the surge of rights doctrines was the declaration of Immanuel Kant in the 1770s that all duties of all humans – including royalty – could be divided into duties of benevolence and duties of justice. With regard to the latter:

> [T]here is no question of inclination, only of the rights of others. It is not their needs that count in this connexion, but their rights; it is not a question of whether my neighbour is needy, wretchedly poor or the reverse; if his right is concerned, it must be satisfied. This group of duties is grounded in the general rule of right [. . . .] The chief of these duties is respect for the rights of others. It is our duty to regard them as sacred and to respect and maintain them as such. There is nothing more sacred in the wide world than the rights of others. They are inviolable (Kant, p.193).

Kant believed that human rights spawned from human reason and free will, not from a God *per se*. However, there was divine inspiration for the construction of a rights-based society since it was the embodiment of God's will "not merely that we should be happy, but that we should make ourselves happy, and this is the true morality" (Kant, p.252). Kant's deontological approach accorded well with most religious moralities, as he emphasized the need to respect the primacy of human life, and the need proactively to help the sick if possible:

> Again, I see a man miserable and I feel for him; but it is useless to wish that he might be rid of his misery; I ought to try to rid him of it (Kant, p.199).

Here we see that Kant has recognized man's duty to help the sick, if possible. It is a duty encumbent upon all people, not only health care professionals (Harris, "Must," p.214). The flip side of this duty – the correlative in Hohfeld's terminology introduced in chapter III – must be a man's right to medical assistance, if available. Rights are, therefore, as stated in chapter III, claims against society, or some segment of it. And the claim to medical assistance, reflected in the duty to provide such assistance, is "almost universally recognized [for] . . . An irreplaceable part of what it is to value life must be a belief that it is better that people live rather than die, and die later rather than earlier and also that their lives be as unimpaired by ill-health, injury, suffering and so on as it is possible to make them" (Harris, *The Value*, p.53).

The balance of this chapter focuses on the considerable complications that arise when the obligation to help others live healthy lives is collectively addressed by a bureaucracy of some sort, as compared to the more straightforward "helping hand" of a neighbor.

Berlin's Polarization and the Power of Negative Thinking

In the middle of the 20th century, Isaiah Berlin analyzed the question of rights as claims against society by viewing such rights as either negative or positive freedoms (he interchangeably uses the term "liberties" as well). Negative freedoms, or liberties, are freedoms from interference by other people with one's own scope of activity (Berlin, p.122). Positive freedoms are freedoms to shape one's own life, including the freedom to participate in shaping the rules that set the ambit of space within which negative liberty reigns (Berlin, p.131). Society has come to admit to an ever-broader array of negative and positive freedoms, and to recognize an ever-greater scope of individual rights. Of these two kinds of rights, however, Berlin emphasizes the supremacy of negative rights because:

> [p]luralism, with the measure of 'negative' liberty that it entails, seems to me a truer and more humane ideal than the goals of those who seek in the great, disciplined, authoritarian structures the ideal of 'positive' self mastery by classes, or peoples, or the whole of mankind (Berlin, p.171).

For example, in the health care field, patients increasingly demand that the government make available new therapies (positive freedom) and ask the government not to interfere with their decisions regarding their own health care (negative freedom). Berlin emphasizes the relatively greater importance of freedom of interference from the government (negative freedom) because:

> it does, at least, recognize the fact that human goals are many, not all of them commensurable . . . . To assume that all values can be graded on one scale, so that it is a mere matter of inspection to determine the highest, seems to me to falsify our knowledge that men are free agents, to represent moral decision as an operation which a slide-rule could, in principle, perform (Berlin, p.171).

Berlin's preference for negative rights may, in fact, become counter-productive in the complex medical ethics arena of the 21st century. Consider the topic of autonomy, a fundamental tenet of medical ethics. Is patient autonomy furthered more by a simple negative proscription against paternalism in medical practice, or by a positive obligation on the part of clinicians to help educate patients as to the nuances of the therapeutic options before them? And if furthered more by the latter, does not such a path also imply an obligation on the part of government to better educate doctors in the area of patient communication, and to affirmatively provide patients with more psycho-social counseling? It can be persuasively demonstrated that patient autonomy, a fundamental right, becomes meaningful for most people only as a critically exercised positive liberty (requiring government involvement in medicine), for otherwise complex decisions devolve into mindlessly-signed informed consent forms.

Notwithstanding Berlin's preferences for negative rights, it is impossible for society to provide health care to masses of people without the government making decisions ostensibly in the public's best interest. In the modern world, the Kantian absolute duty to care for each other's illness is assumed in large part by the State. Not surprisingly, governments argue that budget limitations require them to ration increasingly expensive medical therapies to ensure some optimized level of health care for all. Governments seek in the interests of practical fairness and equality the "slide-rule" that Berlin mocks with disdain. The "slide-rule" creates a conflict between equality and liberty – between society's duty to provide some less expensive health care for all and society's duty to provide greatly needed expensive health care to a few. Berlin summarized this dilemma as follows:

> I do not know who else may have thought this, but it occurred to me that some ultimate values are compatible with each other and some are not. Liberty, in whichever sense, is an eternal human ideal, whether individual or social. So is equality. But perfect liberty (as it must be in the perfect world) is not compatible with perfect equality. If man is free to do anything he chooses, then the strong will crush the weak, the wolves will eat the sheep, and this puts an end to equality (Berlin, *The Power*, p.22).

Berlin's contrapositioning of liberty and equality, makes clear that it is not so simple to fulfill Kant's exhortation to respect rights as "inviolable." The right to health care, for example, may be achieved by some at the expense of many others, or by many others at the expense of a few. Because resources are not infinite, the duty Kant recognized to help "rid a man of his misery," once extrapolated to a national health care system, can devolve into a trade-off between ridding more people of some misery or fewer people of a lot of misery. Hence, while Kant and Hohfeld help us to understand that a right to health care is an individual claim that entails a duty to provide it, Berlin illuminates that in a social system there is no clear-cut answer as to how such a duty might be discharged to those who clamor for scarce goods and services, such as organ transplants. In his classic phrase, "out of the crooked timber of humanity no straight thing was ever made" (Berlin, p.170).

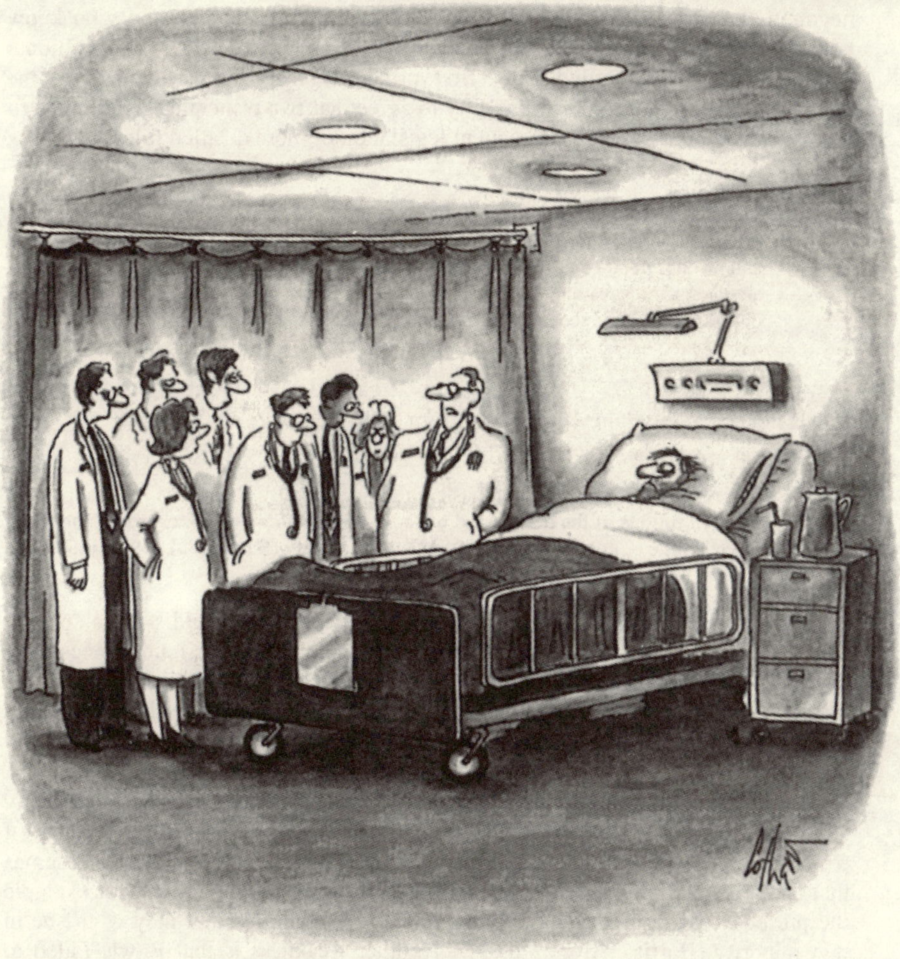

"This patient has a rare form of medical insurance."

Dealing in John Rawls: Primary Goods in a Just Society

The right to an organ transplant fares well under a conceptualization which is focused as much on rectifying differences in equality among a population as it is on the proscription of impingements of negative liberty. Exactly such a novel theory of rights was propounded in 1958 by John Rawls in his essay, *Justice as Fairness* and his 1971 treatise, *A Theory of Justice.*

John Rawls operationalized a contract-like procedure for determining which rights should exist. He did this by imagining a hypothetical constitutional negotiation among humans who know nothing about each other, and who know nothing about their position in the society after the completion of the constitutional negotiation. Rawls argued from first principles that the participants to the negotiation will be forced by rationality to agree that two principles should govern their new society, including subsequent legislation of more detailed rules:

> 1. Each person has an equal right to a fully adequate scheme of equal basic liberties which is compatible with a similar scheme of liberties for all. 2. Social and economic inequalities are to satisfy two conditions. First, they must be attached to offices and positions open to all under conditions of fair equality of opportunity; and second, they must be to the greatest benefit of the least advantaged members of society (Rawls 1987 et al., p.5, 21).

Rawls notes that the rights that evolve from this process are not founded:

> on principles of justice, or on basic (or natural) rights. Rather, its foundation is in the conceptions of the person and of social cooperation most likely to be congenial to the public culture of a modern democratic society (Rawls et al., 1987, p.54).

In other words, if people did not know what their position would be in a society, they would want to ensure that the society could not under any circumstances deny them basic civil and political rights. Furthermore, they would wish to know further that they could not be disenfranchised from opportunities for either social and economic advantage or a fair share of the fruits of such advantages achieved by others.

While the Rawlsian formulation set forth above has won a great many adherents, it has a number of weaknesses. One such weakness is that it presupposes its conclusion. This becomes immediately obvious if one assumes that the persons behind the veil are risk-takers who are willing to risk, for example the presence of a minority slave population, on the gamble that they won't be in that minority (Harris, "More," p.89). Another weakness is that Rawls failed to address the fundamental need for people to enjoy enough health to carry out their contractarian obligations. This oversight is set forth in greater detail below.

Don't Forget About the Health Benefits!

It can be seen that in Rawlsian justice, rights are those primary goods that cannot generally be bartered away and that all people enjoy in equal measure. Consequently, society has a duty to ensure that these rights are exercised without inappropriate infringement. Now, suppose in the original negotiating position posited by Rawls the negotiators thought about their health. A hypothetical discussion might proceed as follows:

Franklin: What about health care? Neither of us would want to be a person in a society who couldn't get great health care, right?

Jefferson: But that implies an inequality, because you may need more health care than I do.

Franklin: Or you may need more than I. If we agree to provide health care for all it will operate to help the least fortunate the most, and is therefore a justifiable inequality.

Jefferson: I think it should be treated as a basic liberty so that people don't trade it away and then get ill. If they don't have the health care they need they will not be healthy enough to exercise even their most basic rights.

In fact, Rawls did not give even this much consideration to the role of health care rights in an original negotiation. He does argue strenuously, though, that self-respect is the most important primary good, and his description of self-respect leaves ample room to extend the right to health care (Rawls 1999, p.386). Determining whether the right to adequate health care can be expanded to include organ transplantation depends upon whether the creation of an adequate supply of organs is (1) compatible with the liberties of others guaranteed by the first Rawlsian principle, and (2) compatible with Rawls' difference principle of only permitting unequal advantages that benefit those who are most disadvantaged. Such details are left by Rawls to legislatures, so Rawls cannot further enlighten us as to the existence of a right to organ transplantation, beyond reading into his theories a right to adequate health care.

Doyal and Gough's Theory of Human Needs

It takes a systematic revision of Rawls to address health care issues such as xenotransplantation concretely, as in a policy-oriented framework. That revision has been offered by Doyal and Gough:

> Rawls' difference principle should be expanded to state that inequalities will only be tolerated to the extent that they benefit the least well off through leading to the provision of those goods and services necessary for the optimisation of basic need-satisfaction (Doyal and Gough, p.132).

By optimization of basic need-satisfaction, Doyal and Gough mean such levels of physical health and personal autonomy as enable people to be minimally disabled in their social participation.

Preeminent among all human needs are the two concerned with physical health and autonomy of agency (Doyal and Gough, p.54). Satisfying the basic needs of physical health and autonomy of agency requires an optimized level of the following intermediate (and readily quantifiable) needs:

1. Food and water
2. Housing
3. Safe work
4. Safe environment
5. Health care
6. Secure childhood
7. Primary relationships
8. Physical security
9. Economic security
10. Safe childbirth
11. Education

Of course, we may have to draw from many different cultural forms in order to satisfy these needs. It is in this way that Doyal and Gough bridge the gap between the universality of basic needs in themselves and the cultural plurality of their appropriate implementation (Doyal and Gough, p.109).

It is one thing to define basic human needs and quite another to demonstrate the existence of a universal right to their satisfaction. While accepting Rawls and Daniels contractarian arguments from rational self-interest, Doyal and Gough demonstrate the inconsistency of imputing moral obligations to others – a fundamental feature of all cultures – without recognition of the right to basic need satisfaction (Doyal and Gough, p.104). They do so through arguing that since ought implies can, the imputation of duties entails the acceptance of the duty to assist in the provision of the necessary goods and services required for the individual and social implementation of those duties (Doyal and Gough, p.104).

> For *without at least minimal levels of need satisfaction, A will be able to do nothing at all, including those acts that are specifically expected of her*. And the same applies to those who believe that they have a right to A's actions. They also must accept that unless her basic needs are minimally satisfied, she will be unable to do what they think she should. Therefore, she has a right to such satisfaction in proportion to the seriousness with which they take her duty and expect her to comply with it (Doyal and Gough, p.94).

It clearly follows from this general argument that all individuals, within any particular culture, have a right to the appropriate health care so that they may best comply with whatever duties of good citizenship are required of them. However, Doyal and Gough provide one further argument to justify the conceptualization of the right to appropriate health care as one that transcends all national boundaries. In their formulation of "critical autonomy" they point out that strongly held beliefs about moral duty in themselves are universal and know no such boundaries (Doyal and Gough, pp.108-09). To this extent, morally committed individuals in the US impute the same moral duties on strangers in foreign countries as they do to their fellow citizens. Using the same logic as has already been described, Doyal and Gough proceed to argue that a universal moral commitment requires the provision of goods and services so that people might choose to conform to it (Doyal and Gough, p.110). Clearly such choices must presuppose in light of the dramatic and potentially traumatic circumstances in which they might occur, the optimal physical health – as well as the education – of the stranger involved. Thus, in short, if individuals in one country wish for all individuals in the world to do what they believe to be right, then they must also be committed to the universal right to appropriate health care.

Why Must My Rights Be Everyone's Rights?

In summary, whereas Rawls does an excellent job of staking out negative rights, his theory of justice is thin in its guidance with regard to positive rights, such as the right to health care. Doyal and Gough strengthen Rawlsian justice with a focus on the basic human need, for health care and autonomy, without which there can be no equal opportunity quest for personal fulfillment. The negative rights protected by Rawls, and the positive health-care rights claimed by patients, both fall into place as crucial enablers of basic human need optimization. *Rawls'* Theory of Justice *and Doyal and Gough's* Theory of Human Need *both, therefore, clearly support a right to health care, and a duty for society to provide it.* This conclusion arises under each of the non-consequentialist avenues for rights generation discussed above: (a) original position negotiations, and (b) human needs analysis.

> a) *Original Position Negotiations* – rights are those claims that negotiators, under a veil of ignorance about each other and their position in a new society, would agree to be available to all members of such a society. Because the negotiators are, in essence, contracting with each other, this approach to rights generation is also called "contractarian." As noted above, the negotiators would surely want to guarantee their ability to access an optimum level of health care, lest they themselves be the sick ones without health care once the veil of ignorance is removed. However, they would not want to provide an unlimited amount of health care to a few extraordinarily sick individuals because, thinking probabilistically, the original position negotiators realize they are unlikely to benefit from such treatment but will have to pay for it. *Consequently, from the*

> *contractarian standpoint, there is a right to an optimum level of health care, subject to available resources.* Furthermore, even total strangers enjoy this right to health care because, behind the "veil of ignorance," we must assume the worst likely case that we could be that stranger.

The fact that "we might be the stranger" is a key reason why one person's right to health care logically must be everyone's right to health care. Very few people would agree to a set of rules for a society in which their ability to receive basic medical care depended on luck, inheritance or wealth. The vast majority of people realize that there is a high probability that under such rules they would be left out. It is a fundamental matter of self-interest to promote universal health care. To the cynic who says "why should I give this health care right to anyone?" there is a simple answer: "you might be anyone" (Ignatieff, p.12). Human rights are a social construct (Gewirth, p.108). It only makes sense to construct something of benefit to oneself. Extrapolated universally, one ends up with a right to health care.

> b) *Human Needs Analysis* – rights are those claims that are necessary in order to perform duties expected of members of a peaceable society. Principally, this includes the achievement of minimally disabled social participation. One cannot perform the roles of an active citizen, or of a person fulfilling their personal ambitions to the best of their ability, if one cannot be made healthy (if possible) when one is disabled. Consequently, execution of the normal duties expected of a member of society implies an obligation on the part of society to provide its members with a reasonable level of health care. Keeping with Hohfeldian correlatives, there must be a right to health care because society has a duty to provide for the health of its members, to the extent that societal resources are available.

The fact that we live in societies in which we are highly interdependent on other people is a second key reason why there is a right to health care. If we did not vest this right in everyone, then we would begin to feel the cost of others' unrequited illness or through the interdependencies of social life. The illnesses of others spread illness to us, and the absence of others leaves us without workers, customers and professional services. At times, people imagine that they are immune from these problems, but soon enough interdependencies snap into place like a web of rubber bands. Schools close, trains stop, business dries up, and, worst of all, illness spreads. Nothing less than the instinct for social survival relentlessly drives societies toward recognizing that the human need for basic health care must be met. Consequently, enlightened self interest ensures that the right to health care is not jealously guarded by a few, but instead – sooner or later – is made available to all. As Jonathan Mann observed in 1994:

> The proposal that promoting and protecting human rights is inextricably linked to the challenge of promoting and protecting health derives in part from recognition that health and human rights are complementary approaches to the central problem of defining and advancing human well-being (Mann 1994, p.19).

It should be reemphasized that this right to health care is neither absolute nor a governmental guarantee of a person's good health. The latter extreme is "obviously absurd." Instead, the right should be construed as one that guarantees medical treatment and healthy conditions that evolve with time and technology (Leary, pp.28, 31). It is also important to summarize the benefits of rights-based conceptualizations – for which the underpinnings have been provided by Rawls (as what would arise from original position negotiations), as compared to the non-rights-based utilitarian theories described earlier:

1) Conceptualizing something as a right emphasizes its exceptional importance as a social or public goal (rights as "trumps")
2) Rights concepts focus on the dignity of persons
3) Equality of non-discrimination is a fundamental principle of human rights
4) Participation of individuals and groups in issues affecting them is an essential aspect of human rights
5) The concept of rights implies entitlement
6) Rights are interdependent
7) Rights are almost never absolute and may be limited, but such limitations should be subject to strict scrutiny (Leary, p.46).

Whether needs-generated or contractarian-generated, the right to health care does not necessarily imply *a right to an organ transplant.* The existence of such a particularized right, as part and parcel of the right to health care, depends in part upon the availability of xenotransplantation in order for the needed organs to even be available. In addition, however, whether there is a right to an organ transplant will depend upon whether xenotransplantation:

a) helps to optimize health care by extending life to millions of people dying of end stage organ failure;
b) or actually puts it in jeopardy by diverting resources from other health care programs or spreading new zoonoses.

Giving an Inch and Taking a Mile: Can Health Care Include Xenotransplantation?

Doyal and Gough have written extensively on the meaning of "health" and the delimitation of what constitutes "access to health care." A review of their conceptions should prove valuable in order to determine whether the right to health care includes a specific right to xenotransplantation. They pointedly observe that:

> survival is, so to speak, the bottom line of the need for physical health. Unless individuals are alive, they do not even have the chance of becoming ill, much less of doing anything else . . . . We have argued that individuals have a right of access to the means to survival to the degree that they are physically capable of it . . . . Yet persons are also deprived if their survival chances are artificially limited by social and economic circumstances which are alterable (Doyal and Gough, p.172).

Transplantation in general is, and xenotransplantation will be, of course, medical technology of last resort; in other words, "the means to survival." The risks of organ rejection and surgical mishap are so life threatening that transplantation procedures are not even considered until all else has failed or is failing. Consequently, it seems clear that a right of access to health care includes a right of access to xenotransplantation technology, both for those who need it, and subject to any other considerations of a resource limitation or public health concern nature. This conclusion is made even more manifest by a consideration of the measurable parameters Doyal and Gough have suggested as indicators of basic need-satisfaction for:

Basic Need Component	**Suggested Indicators**
Physical health	
Survival chances	Life expectancy at various ages
	Age-specific mortality rates; infant mortality
Physical ill-health	Prevalence of disabilities, by severity
	Frequency of child development deficiencies
	Prevalence of people suffering serious pain
	Morbidity rates for various diseases

(Doyal and Gough, p.190)

Looking at these indicators adds yet further ammunition to xenotransplantation's standing as a *bona fide* candidate for any right to health care. With regard to the basic need sub-component of "survival chances," approximately one-third of all people die from organ failure. Xenotransplantation would directly improve life expectancy, especially in the later decades of life. Furthermore, the organ gap is considered widest for children and neonates – harvested human organs are overwhelmingly from adults and too large for children. Xenografts could be made available in various sizes and would constitute a tremendous resource for pediatric transplantation.

As to the basic need sub-component of "physical ill-health," numerous disabilities, development deficiencies, causes of serious pain, and chronic morbidities are traceable to organ failure. For example, the disability, developmental deficiency (for children) and agonizing morbidity of dialysis for kidney failure would be eliminated with a robust supply of kidney xenografts. The incapacitation and frightful pain of chronic heart disease would be resolved with a robust supply of transplantable pig hearts. The developmental deficiencies and debilitating morbidity of lung diseases such as cystic fibrosis and a wide variety of liver diseases would be sharply reduced with an ample supply of transplantable porcine lungs and livers, respectively. On the other hand, transplantation itself introduces illness (e.g., rejection) and may not completely ameliorate preexisting illnesses (e.g., Cystic Fibrosis).

Xenotransplantation cannot reasonably be looked at as some kind of a "luxury therapy" which is unnecessary for materially enhancing physical health. More people in the West die of heart disease than any other condition, and organ failure is the proximate cause of most pediatric deaths in the West. For these millions of persons xenotransplantation, if available, means survival. For many additional millions it means elimination of social participation blocking morbidities.

No Religious Preference

An interesting perspective on the transculturality of the right to transplantation technology can be gleaned from a case study exercise undertaken by the European Network of Scientific Co-operation on Medicine and Human Rights. In Case 78, a "hospital service refuses hemodialysis or inclusion on the waiting list for renal transplants for a man of 71 suffering from an evolutive bilateral renal sclerosis, budgetary considerations imposing other priorities" (European Network of Scientific Co-operation on Medicine and Human Rights, p.366).

An expert on Muslim ethics assessed Case 78 as follows:

> To refuse hemodialysis for a 71-year-old patient is shocking, to put it mildly. Furthermore, the budgetary problem cannot be a reason for not including him on the waiting list for a renal transplant. The Koran (Sura II, v.211) recommends succouring one's neighbour, and Sura V, v. 32, states that "He who saveth a life, shall be as though he had saved all mankind alive" (European Network of Scientific Co-operation on Medicine and Human Rights, pp.368-69).

Remarkably similar was the view from the standpoint of Jewish ethics:

> It is inadmissible to discriminate between citizens and have a two-tier medical system. Every person has a right to the health care he needs. It is inadmissible that budgetary reasons should lead to the refusal to treat a patient. Budgetary reasons may never be invoked when a human life is at stake. To allow this is once again to open the door to all the abuses. Tomorrow, there will be no more care for old people, and after that it may be the turn of immigrants and foreigners, etc. This patient of 71 should be admitted to the hospital service and given the dialysis he needs. He should also be added to the waiting list for renal transplants if the conditions required for this transplant are fulfilled (European Network of Scientific Co-operation on Medicine and Human Rights, p.368).

Also in accord was the Buddhist view: The patient's age does not justify his being denied the benefit of modern techniques which could help him (European Network of Scientific Co-operation on Medicine and Human Rights, p.369).

Conclusion

Does the right to an optimum level of medical care include xenotransplantation? The answer is a qualified yes, qualified by budgetary and public health constraints. Because xenotransplantation is a life-saving and morbidity reducing technology, States have an obligation to encourage its development. And, once it is shown to be safe and effective, States have an obligation to make it available to all persons on an equitable, non-discriminatory basis – if the State can afford to make it available at all. Consequently, humans do have a right to have safe xenotransplantation technology developed and made available to them in accordance with budgetary constraints. All of this, however, is subject to the caveat that the public health is not in fact jeopardized by xenotransplantation. It is to this issue that the next chapter is addressed.

Chapter VI

Is Xenotransplantation Worth the Risk?

The preceding chapter concluded with an overriding sense that there is a compelling right to xenotransplantation. This right is borne of society's obligation to provide optimal satisfaction of the human need for health. Notwithstanding the strength of a xenotransplantation right, it is not absolute. The right is penned in by the proviso that its exercise be consistent with *public* health. The rights of the individual do not always trump the interests of the collective. In a health care context, this is evident in that even the near-sacrosanct right to confidentiality, which harkens back to Hippocrates, may be superceded, if necessary for the protection of public health. Consequently, it falls to this chapter to assess how much risk is appropriate to impose on the community for the good of the individual. The reciprocal question is equally vital: how much risk of ill health is appropriate to impose on the individual to assuage the public health fears of the community?

Introduction

Twice before, society has grappled with questions analogous to xenotransplantation. In the 1940s, society decided to unleash antibiotics into the ecosphere of human and animal health, with full knowledge that doing so breeds new bacteria against which humanity may lack adequate defenses. The feared risk occurred, and today *tens of thousands of people die each year* as a result of antibiotic-resistant infectious diseases. Even though this sounds equivalent to the speculated harm from xenogeneic-spawned zoonoses, there is no general clamor for banning or even severely restricting antibiotics. To this day, antibiotics ethics revolves around the question of whether the needs of a few have jeopardized the well-being of many – does the antibiotics experience teach us the extent to which the individual right to health care can trump the public health interests of the collective, or are there other explanations? For example, is a much more prohibitive regime appropriate for xenotransplantation because it risks creating *new* diseases whereas antibiotic resistance arises from efforts to manage *old* diseases?

More recently, in the 1980s, recombinant DNA research and products were approved for development and use. Scientists were permitted to use cancer-causing viruses to convey new DNA into cultured human cells, even though this posed a non-dismissable risk of creating new infectious forms of cancer. Here, too, the risks of creating dangerous new microbial life forms were balanced against the benefits of forging powerful new medicines. Recombinant DNA ethics places great emphasis on the detailed regulatory and technological precautions that have been adopted to guard against inadvertent creation of new diseases. However, no one claims the risk is zero. Does the recombinant DNA experience demonstrate the strength, or the feebleness, of public health concerns as a counter-balance to freedom of scientific research and the right to health care? The debates over antibiotics and recombinant DNA will help shed light on the ethically most appropriate course to follow in the realm of xenotransplantation technology.

Truth or Consequences: Incommensurability of Negativities

A conceptual problem with risk assessment lies with what Nicholas Rescher calls the "incommensurability of negativities."

> To assess and compare risks we must be in a position to measure them so as to determine the extent of their relative overall seriousness. And this requires us to be in a position to assess and compare the size of various negativities. Unfortunately, however, there is no assurance that different negativities can be measured in a common comparability unit – that they all have a mutually commensurable quantitative size. The very idea of the relative magnitude of negativities is problematic . . . . And the situation becomes yet murkier when the quantitative aspects of degree, diffusion, and timing are brought on the stage. Thus, how is one to trade off greater intensity and less diffusion against lesser intensity and more diffusion, or greater immediacy and lesser intensity against lesser immediacy and higher intensity, or the like (Rescher, p.20).

One might think that a comparison can be made by reducing the various risks such as immediate mortality due to lack of a xenograft or possible future morbidity due to incapacitation with a xenogeneic virus to lost man-hours or dollars. However, a simplified numerical example from Rescher shows that such "incommensurability of negativities" can easily result in a counter-intuitive outcome that most people would not accept:

> Negativity #1: the death of two children with an average future life expectancy of 70 years.
>
> Negativity #2: the incapacitation (say by a serious bout of influenza) of 16,000 people for an average period of 4 days.
>
> With negativity #1, the man-day loss stands at 2x70x365=51,000 man-days, with negativity #2, the man-day loss is 16,000x4=64,000. Yet it is surely far from clear that #1 is preferable to #2 (Rescher, p.21).

The incommensurability of negativities makes the classic risk assessment algorithm seem to be little more than a forced construction of the risk assessor's reality upon an inherently ambiguous reality. Nevertheless, as with ethical analysis itself, if risk assessment is used to analyze and clarify a situation, rather than dictate a mandatory result, it can be a useful tool. Rescher teaches avoidance of simplistic numerical formulas as substitutes for the complexities of risk assessment.

> There just is no automatic process for balancing a severe loss for few against a minor loss for many, say by equating a 10% disability of 50 people with a 100% disability of 5. And exactly the same sort of story holds for the other parametric components of hazard . . . . It is a fundamental and far-reaching fact of risk analysis that the different parameters of negativity are not necessarily commensurable. ... Any attempt to measure this 'size' of a negativity by a single number derived from some assumed common denominator involves the problematic oversimplification of an inherently complex picture (Rescher, p.21).

For example, there is no objective means of balancing a certain million deaths a year due to lack of xenografts against possible new pandemic xenoviruses that may cause flu-like illness, or perhaps even early death. Consequently, the countless variables involved in assessing xenotransplantation risk are so immeasurable, incomparable and unique that it constitutes a classic example of the incommensurability of negativities.

Garbage In, Garbage Out: Inestimability of Probabilities

In addition to the "mind-game" nature of comparing incomparable harms, a further impediment stands in the way of classical risk analysis for xenotransplantation: it is tremendously difficult to estimate the *probability of harm* from xenogeneic viruses. This handicap on the second term in the risk assessment algorithm arises from the impossibility of estimating what any life form, including any virus in existence today, will look like in the future, let alone the probability that it will remain harmless. For example, quite recently a new porcine zoonosis jumped to humans, much as occurred in the swine flu epidemic – without any involvement from xenotransplantation. In "1998-89 the Malaysian Nipah virus, causing viral encephalitis, jumped from pigs to humans, infected 269 people, killed over 100, left dozens brain damaged, and led to the mass slaughter of one million pigs" (Fano et al., p.869). Yet, it would be absurd to propose isolating humans from farm animals. Some risk of zoonoses is inherent to life on earth. The crucial question is does the *new medium of transmission* involved in xenotransplantation *meaningfully increase* the zoonotic threat to public health above and beyond that which already exists? And, if so, are the potential benefits worth the increased risk?

Recall from chapter III that to date *no* zoonoses have arisen from xenotransplantation, although the only surgeries which patients survived long-term are the xenografting of porcine pancreatic islet cells and the xenoperfusion of a patient's blood through porcine livers. Also, pig farmers and butchers "who most frequently expose themselves to pig tissue through cuts on their hands," have not shown any greater likelihood of contracting diseases from their pigs or other animals (Cooper and Lanza, p.164). These facts argue against a meaningful increase in zoonoses due to xenotransplantation, although the experience is of course limited.

How "small a risk" is "small enough" to warrant new biotechnological developments? On the one hand, the answer to this question depends on the kind of harm risked. We are less willing to risk a pandemic harm than a localized one. However, when multiplied against pandemic risks, some very small risks will be assigned an effectively zero probability because, were they not, they would stop highly desired actions from occurring. Even very small numbers, when multiplied by very, *very* large negative numbers, produce large negative numbers. For example, there is some risk that if greenhouse gases are not halted immediately then the polar caps will melt and most of the world's population will die in massive floods. This risk is assigned by nearly everyone an effective zero probability because, were it not, the actions required to off-set the risk would fundamentally alter society (e.g., a dramatic reduction in the use of the internal combustion engine).

Humanity tends to follow the precept *de minimis non curat lex (there is no need to bother with trifles)*. In physical systems, there is something called "background noise" which can be ignored without sacrificing valid computations. Reschler has noted that "in deliberating about risks to human life, for example, there is some tendency to take as a baseline the chance of death by natural disasters (or "acts of God"), roughly 1/1,000,000 per annum in the USA" (Rescher, p.37). The "background noise" for xenogeneic viruses is the natural zoonoses that occur from time to time, like influenza epidemics, HIV and the Malaysian Nipah virus, combined with other man-made disease threats. Consequently, from the standpoint of the probability prong of the risk assessment algorithm, it could be asked, "Does xenotransplantation pose more than a one in a million chance of causing death above and beyond that caused by other infectious disease causes, or is it just part of this 'background noise' threat to humanity?" While such a question does help to focus and clarify the risk assessment issues involved, it is also inherently unanswerable.

Because of the "incomparability of negativities" and the "inestimability of probabilities, it is indeed difficult to quantify the meaning of risk. However, as will be seen below, important lessons can be learned from case studies of antibiotics and recombinant DNA. In the case of antibiotics, it will be shown that the world "messed up" – antibiotic-resistant pathogens are now a serious, epidemic-threatening global problem costing thousands of lives each year. However, in the case of recombinant DNA, the world seems to have "got it right." Risk-minimization policies have enabled twenty years of gene splicing to occur without deaths. In this chapter we will study what was wrong with antibiotics policy and what was right about recombinant DNA policy, in light of the similar lack of predictability of the pandemic risk of xenotransplantation. In the following chapter we will apply the lessons learned from these debates to ensure a safe introduction of xenotransplantation technology.

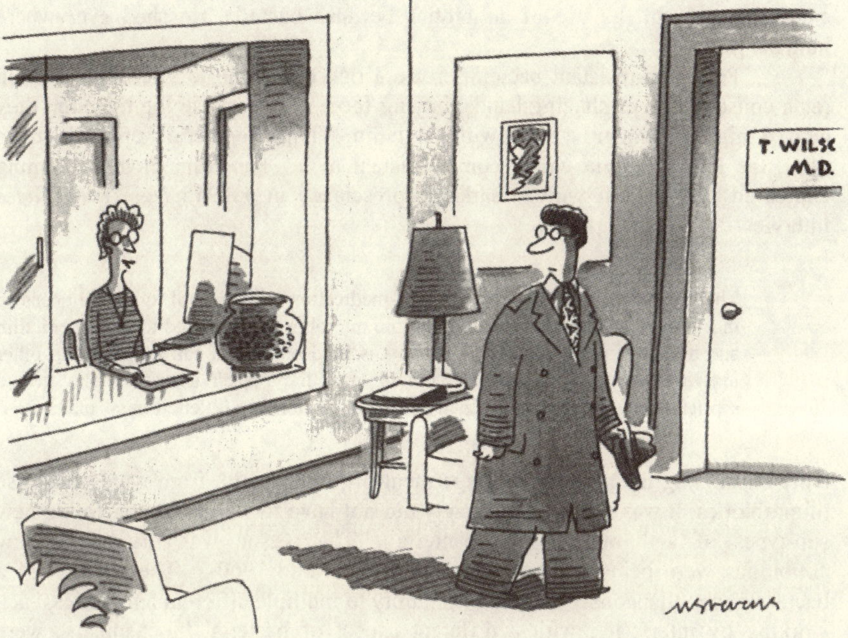

"Don't forget to take a handful of our complimentary antibiotics on your way out."

Antibiotics: Better Not Sorry Than Safe

Antibiotics entered into medical use in the 1930s (sulpha drugs) and 1940s (penicillin). By trial and error, researchers discovered that these drugs dramatically reduced the morbidity and mortality associated with a wide variety of conditions caused by harmful bacteria. These and other antibiotics initially killed various types of harmful (and harmless and helpful) bacteria they encountered. Claims were made that thousands, or even millions, of lives had been saved by antibiotics (Wainwright, p.10). More than 2000 tons of the relatively toxic suphonamide drugs were used by 1941, and 17,000 tons of penicillin were used annually by 1980 (Cannon, p.57).

As early as 1940, it was already recognized that, over time, bacteria became resistant to specific antibiotics. This was understood even by penicillin pioneer Alexander Fleming to be the consequence of Darwinian natural selection at the breakneck pace of bacterial reproduction. In any population of billions of bacteria there is a probability of a genetic mutation that renders a single bacterium invincible to the biochemical harm inflicted by a particular antibiotic. That single bacterium will multiply and all the others will die. Very soon, the bacterial colony will be resistant to the antibiotic that was once effective against it because the colony will be comprised of a mutated variant of the original bacteria. This was a cautionary tale in the use of antibiotics because bacteria are shed everywhere humans go.

Penicillin-resistant bacteria create a risk to anyone to whom they attach (as a consequence of shaking hands, buying food, etc.) because the infection they caused might no longer be cured with penicillin. The more liberally an antibiotic is used, the more bacteria will become resistant to it. Penicillin pioneer Fleming expressed his concern with remarkable prescience in a 1945 *New York Times* interview.

> The greatest possibility of evil in self-medication is the use of too small doses so that instead of clearing up infection, the microbes are educated to resist penicillin and a host of penicillin-fast organisms is bred out which can be passed to other individuals and from them to others until they reach someone who gets a septicemia or a pneumonia which penicillin cannot save ("Pencillin's," p.21).

Notwithstanding the possible endangerment of public health from widespread use of antibiotics, it was argued that society did not have to worry about creating new sub-types of antibiotic-resistant bacteria. The reason was that many new antibiotics were being synthesized in the 1950s and 1960s. The chances of a bacterium simultaneously mutating immunity to multiple different antibiotics, each working by interfering with a different aspect of bacterial biochemistry, were considered infinitesimal. Consequently, scientists and policy-makers assured themselves in the 1950s that the public health risks of liberal use of antibiotics were outweighed by the benefits of such use since bacterial adaptation could always be outsmarted with new generations of antibiotics.

As a result, the use of antibiotics burgeoned beyond the prescription slip to include prophylactic use against gonorrhea by soldiers and prostitutes in Vietnam, aerosol spraying of entire buildings that housed sick people, consumer bathroom products, unregulated sales in developing countries as "cure-alls," and mass dousing of factory-farmed animals. In a span of just a few decades humans created entire new species of antibiotic resistant bacteria which today dominate their microbial ancestors, i.e., most harmful bacteria in the world are now impervious to the antibiotic traditionally used against them.

> We can no longer expect that any infection will be cured by the first antibiotic chosen. In some parts of the world, limited supplies of antibiotics mean that no available antibiotic is effective. This is a far cry from the situation just twenty

> years ago. Resistance takes its toll in deaths where newer antibiotics are unavailable or in patients in whom an antibiotic's side effects precludes its use. Patients are suffering and dying from diseases that some predicted forty years ago would be wiped off the face of the earth (Levy, p.11).

The Institute of Medicine conducted a workshop on microbial resistance that specifically quantified an example of the differential, detrimental effect of antibiotic resistance. The workshop noted, that due to the liberal use of antibiotics more than 90 percent of *Staphylococcus aureus* strains are resistant to the usual treatment, methicillin. In New York City, in 1995, methicillin-resistant infections represented 29 percent of the incidence of all nosocomial infections but 48 percent of mortality from such infections (Institute of Medicine 1998, p.11). Methicillin-susceptible *S. aureus* infections had an 8 percent mortality compared to a 17 percent mortality for methicillin-resistant infections. Clearly, the introduction of antibiotics to help some people has caused others to lose their lives. The situation is remarkably similar to the fear that xenotransplantation for the benefit of some will result in xenogeneic diseases to the detriment of others.

In the early 1950s, Dr. Tsutomo Watanabe discovered bacteria that were resistant to more than one antibiotic. He further proved that this was caused by the transfer of resistance genes (originated as a result of random mutation in a particular bacterium) from one colony of bacteria to another colony, and even across different species of bacteria. *This was devastating news because it meant that bacteria effectively were "learning" from one another; their capabilities were no longer limited by Darwinian principles.* Indeed, natural selection was now seen to be operating upon bacteria that *acquired* characteristics not only through mutations in their own colony, but through transference of resistance capability from mutations in other colonies. Antibiotics expert Richard Novick, summarized the reaction as follows:

> Appalled by the implications, [I] wrote letters to the *Lancet* warning against the then common practice of surgeons in London hospitals, of "spraying methicillin around the wards. I wrote saying this was outrageous, and would ruin the usefulness of the drug." So it proved, with the emergence of MRSA – methicillin-resistant *S. Aureus* (Cannon, p.188).

By the 1960s, scientists realized that bacteria contain small circles of genetic material in addition to their single chromosome. These circles, called "plasmids," replicate within the bacterial cell walls, and copies can be passed to another bacteria of an entirely different type when the two are in physical contact. Hence, a plasmid mutation that protects against antibiotic A in bacteria X, can be transferred to bacteria Y, which may already benefit from a plasmid mutation that protects against antibiotic B. Keeping in mind that people have trillions of bacteria within their bodies, and there are countless additional bacteria on all things touched by people (and plants and animals), it is easy to see how bacteria can evolve that are resistant to all antibiotics. Simply put, the more antibiotics that a bacteria is resistant to, the more likely it is to multiply and thrive in an environment where less-resistant bacteria are being killed off by one antibiotic or another. In 1967, Dr. Watanabe warned the world that "unless we put a halt to the prodigal use of antibiotics and synthetic drugs, we may soon be forced back into the pre-antibiotic era of medicine" (Watanabe, p.19).

Acquired resistance clearly requires a sharp reassessment of the public health ramifications of antibiotics. The use of antibiotics to help people who are suffering from a non-self-limited infection, or who want to avoid serious infection as a consequence of surgery, creates a risk of creating a "superbug" that causes a global pandemic (Cannon, p.175). Such a pandemic could be caused by the transfer of antibiotic resistance genes from plasmids to a common bacteria, that via mutation, develops virulent characteristics. For example, *E. coli* blankets human gastrointestinal tracts and is generally harmless. However, a virulent form of *E. coli* could arise via random mutation. Ordinarily, doctors would treat the harmful bacteria with antibiotics. But if the harmful variant of *E. coli* acquired antibiotic resistance genes via plasmid transfer, then medical science would have no weapon to use against it (Cannon, p.175). In this way, the widespread use of antibiotics has put the entire human population at risk.

The actual death toll from antibiotic resistance is becoming significant, although different sets of assumptions result in varying estimates:

- One expert, Professor Alexander Tomasz of Rockefeller University in New York, reckoned in 1994 that deaths from hospital infections in the USA, mostly involving drug resistant bacteria, totaled 65,000-70,000 a year (Cannon, p.171).
- A workshop report on antimicrobial resistance by the prestigious U.S. Institute of Medicine, reported that antibiotic-resistant bacteria generate a minimum of $4 billion to $5 billion in costs to U.S. society and individuals yearly, and the 19,000 deaths directly caused by hospital-acquired infections made them the eleventh leading cause of death in the U.S. population (Institute of Medicine 1998, pp.9-10).

Further upping the ante on endangerment of public health is the widespread use of antibiotics in animal husbandry. A tabulation of this use, degree of overuse (i.e., unambiguous misuse) and the resultant new microbe variants is provided in the Table below. Even without xenotransplantation, antibiotic practices alone cause increasingly harmful zoonoses to appear in man simply because the use of antibiotics in animals renders existing zoonoses antibiotic-resistant. After reviewing several studies that demonstrated the transference of antibiotic resistance traits into humans via the consumption of antibiotic treated animals, one expert concluded:

> the use of antibiotics as feed additives creates potential for a reservoir of transferable resistance determinants. A permanent communication between this reservoir and reservoirs in the human body (above all the intestinal flora) is maintained with the food chain as the main route of transmission . . . . Although it is difficult to quantify the extent of this spread, antibiotic use in animal feeding obviously contributes to the development of resistance in human bacterial pathogens (Witte, p.69).

Antibiotic practices create new diseases in people worldwide because the use of antibiotics transforms existing bacterial diseases into antibiotic-resistant bacterial diseases (Levy, p.205). Consequently, the risk of creating new infectious diseases in man cannot automatically "blackball" a new medical technology. After all, antibiotic practices not only risk creating new infectious diseases in man; they actually have done so.

Table VI-1 Estimated Annual Antimicrobial Use in Humans and Animals in the United States, and Resistant Pathogens

Use/Site	Amount	Misuse	Major Resistant Pathogens
Humans/ Hospital	190 M doses/day	25-45%	Staphylococci, enterococci gram-negative rods
Humans/ Community	145 M doses/day	20-50%	Pneumococci, gonococci, Group A streptococci, Escherichia coli, Mycobacterium Tuberculosis
Animals/ Farms	20 Million pounds yr	40-80%	Salmonella, Campylobacter

(Source: Institute of Medicine 1998, pp.40-41)

We Tolerate the Risks for the Sake of the Benefits

Antibiotics are an example of a conflict between public and private interests in healthcare. They impose risk on the society (because recovering patients shed, excrete and otherwise spread around town their surviving antibiotic resistant bacteria) at the same time as they help save the lives of individual members of society. The question to ask is, why does society permit the widespread use of antibiotics given the endangerment such use poses to public health? In a nutshell, the public is willing to tolerate a currently known harm (a significant, steady but not dramatically increasing death toll), and risk even greater harm (a resistant bacteriological pandemic or epidemics), because of reasoned arguments regarding the benefits of antibiotics (many lives saved and made less painful), and confidence that public health regulations could always solve any alarmingly harmful situation "in real time." In a similar vein, the public can be expected to tolerate xenotransplantation risks if the benefits are tangible and if the risks appear to be manageable.

Benefits are Great. Part of the reason the public thinks antibiotics are so great is as a result of the "miracle drug" *imprimatur* the media gave to penicillin in the midst of World War II (Levy, pp.41-42). Over half a century later, it will not be easy to take back something that the public has become so accustomed to thinking of as a cure, even if its effect is usually that of a placebo at best, and a hidden danger at worst. The popularity of antibiotics also extends to the 50 percent of all antibiotics that are used in animal husbandry because farmers are a powerful lobby. They advocate for antibiotics in order to improve animal economics (Levy, p.141). Fortunately, some countries have been able to reduce the amount of antibiotics used on animals by prohibiting subtherapeutic uses (Levy, p.142). Remaining therapeutic uses, however, still generate countless billions of antibiotic-resistant potentially zoonotic bacteria. But this risk is accepted because the public believes that the benefits of antibiotics are worth the risks of harm.

Risks Appear Manageable. The public may also be reasoning that the benefits outweigh the risks of antibiotics because the risks have not yet seemed alarming or dramatic. For decades, experts have been warning of antibiotic-generated "superbugs" that pose pandemic threats to human society. However, the threat has, to date, materialized in relatively limited forms:

- thousands of lives were lost in Central America in the 1970s due to multiresistant *Shigella* bacteria, but Central American lives lost to diarrhea do not figure prominently in Euro-American policymaking;

- hundreds of lives lost to a 1980s epidemic in Zaire of multiresistant *Shigella dysenteriae* did not seem threatening to the West, or unusual given Zaire's numerous causes of premature death;

- an "Imminent Hazard" petition submitted to the U.S. Secretary of Health and Human Services in 1985 asking for an animal use ban on antibiotics based on the growing number of *Salmonella* deaths was rejected based on an alleged lack of evidence for "imminence of hazard";

- tetracycline resistant strains of *V. cholerae* that now plague large parts of Africa are viewed more as diseases of poverty than of antibiotic resistance;

- outbreaks of multiply resistant *Staphylococcus aureus* have largely been limited to hospitals, and have been shown to be containable with isolation strategies (Levy, 202);

- the tens of thousands of Euro-American lives lost to multiple-resistant hospital acquired infections, mostly pneumonia are perceived as inevitable diseases of the very young, very old, or immunosuppressed.

While each of these "limited" instances of antibiotic-generated death and disability are ominous warning signs, none of them have the frightening characteristics of an imminent plague. There is no "clear and present danger" for government to use as a lever to change entrenched antibiotic consumption practices. Experts warn policymakers to curtail antibiotics now before there is a plague, but policymakers rarely heed expert warnings about possible future dangers. Furthermore, experts also have found that an antibiotic resistance predominance can be overturned if antibiotics are removed (Lenski, p.133). The reversal takes much more time to occur than does the establishment of resistance (during which much death or disability can occur in society) (Lenski, p.132). And the reversal tends to take longer and longer if resistant strains are kept in place by constant antibiotic use (Lenski, p.139). Nevertheless, the very possibility of such a resistance reversal provides confidence that a regulatory solution will be available if and when it is needed.

Benefits Outweigh Risks. In 1900, "three bacterial diseases – tuberculosis, pneumonia and diarrhoeal disease – were the leading causes of death, accounting for almost 30% of mortality" (Cohen, "Epidemiological," p.223). While better public health practices eliminated much of this toll in developed countries, "for many infectious diseases, antimicrobial agents were the key factor in decreasing both morbidity and mortality by curtailing transmission among the general public and reducing the complications of infectious diseases for the individual patient" (Cohen, "Epidemiological," p.224). The benefits appear to outweigh the costs, especially when it is said that the costs can be reduced yet further by reasonable regulatory practices and technology developments such as:

- More prudent use of antibiotics; and
- Development of new antibiotics.

Since the risk society is willing to assume is relative to the expected benefits, and the benefits of antibiotics appear to be dramatic, society is willing to assume even the risks of new antibiotic-spawned pandemic diseases. Supporting society's willingness to assume this risk is the sense that while the potential harm is enormous, the likelihood of such potential harm actually occurring is small. Furthermore, these low probability risks can be rendered even less onerous with reasonable regulations (Levy, p.243).

The first analogy of this chapter, antibiotics and microbial resistance, provides an answer to one of the two questions posed at the beginning of the chapter: "*what is meant* by *unacceptable endangerment* of public health?" The answer is a perception that the *harm* causable by a new medical technology is *greater* than the benefits it delivers. Since the harm caused by antibiotics is perceived to be of a *lesser* magnitude than its benefits, antibiotic technology is accepted. Applying the experience to xenotransplantation, it may be concluded that its acceptance will be directly tied to its demonstrated ability to deliver meaningful benefits and to the perceived ability of a regulatory scheme to manage xenogeneic risks. A major question is whether the risks of xenotransplantation *can* be throttled. In other words, we are now faced with the second question raised at the beginning of this chapter: *how does one know* that the risk of harm has been rendered acceptable? The next section answers this question by taking an in-depth look at recombinant DNA technology.

Containing Pandora: Russian Doll Treatment of Recombinant DNA

The very plasmid-delivered DNA that so worried those fighting bacteriological resistance (because they transferred genes from one kind of bacterium to another), was a holy grail to another group of life scientists. This latter group of biologists saw in plasmids a way to convey new DNA into a cell, thereby changing its genetic nature. Ironically, the bane of one sub-discipline of life scientists (who largely called themselves "microbiologists") became the paradigm of another sub-discipline (who rallied under the rubric "molecular biologists").

In the early 1970s, molecular biologists developed techniques to splice genes from long chromosomes of one organism and insert them into the chromosomes of another organism, often using plasmids as "vector." These techniques became known as "genetic engineering" and the resultant product was called "recombinant DNA." In fact, cellular chimeras were being created. Proponents of this technology speculated that genetic engineering could be used to increase food production (e.g., frost-resistance genes could be spliced into produce that are often lost to frost), and to make new medicines (e.g., genes to make scarce biomolecules could be spliced into the chromosomes of harmless bacteria thereby turning them into bio-factories for new medicines). Opponents feared that harmful laboratory bacteria would get recombinant DNA that allowed them to penetrate the human ecosystem and create new pandemic diseases.

In the 1970s, the biggest question hanging over the head of genetic engineering was "how does society know whether or not endangerment of public health will occur?" Consequently, the National Academy of Sciences organized a meeting to answer this question. The invitees included scientific experts from several countries, a few lawyers with experience in bioethics, and media observers. The meeting was held the week of February 24th, 1975, at the Asilomar Conference Center in Pacific Grove, California. The tasks of the meeting were to: (1) discuss the risks of recombinant DNA research, (2) embody any consensus in a public statement, and (3) submit a comprehensive report regarding what to do about such risks to the Academy. This meeting, now known as Asilomar in biotechnology lore, concluded that *there was no way to know* whether or not well-meaning genetic engineering experiments could produce unanticipated, malevolent results – ranging from cancer in lab workers to new infectious diseases. As a result, for the first time in history, a group of scientists imposed upon themselves restrictions as to what kinds of experiments could be done, and under what kinds of laboratory conditions. These procedures are now followed worldwide. Today, there are many agricultural and medicinal products born of recombinant DNA. No new diseases have been created.

The recombinant DNA experience may provide a good precedent of how to ethically address the possible risks to public health of xenotransplantation. As with genetic engineering, the biggest question with xenografts is how does society know whether it is creating a new risk to public health? As discussed in chapter III, there is no way to know for sure whether or not a new disease will be borne of xenotransplantation. In essence, when the very existence of a major risk is difficult to discern, it is wise to take every reasonable precaution to isolate that risk, but not to quash the research that gives rise to the risk in the first place – for to quash the risk would also be to quash its beneficial potential.

The foregoing risk assessment calculus is well-summarized in Reschler's three cardinal rules of risk-taking:

I. Maximize Expected Values

II. Avoid Catastrophes

III. Dismiss Extremely Remote Possibilities

Rescher notes that the rules must be prioritized in reverse order to produce results which match with everyday experience:

> (III) takes precedence over (II), which in turn takes precedence over (I) . . . . First, catastrophe is seen to represent an unacceptable risk, when "the game's not worth the candle" because the potential negative outcomes, unlikely though their realization may be, are simply too massive for the stakes otherwise at issue. But, secondly, this principle itself needs to be curtailed, when it becomes too conservative in its operation and leads to a stultification of action. Just this rationale motivates the recourse to "effective zero" probabilities. Such an analysis indicates that even the "rational man" will refuse to adopt an unqualified and uncompromising expected-value approach to assessing the acceptability of risks (Rescher, pp.117-18).

In essence, as will be seen below, society first applied Rule II, found it likely to lead to "stultification" and thus adopted a set of risk containment procedures that, if followed religiously, redefined the risk as one covered by Rule III. Once that was done, the expected values of recombinant DNA technology could be realized.

The Asilomar Story

In the early 1970s, a class of "restriction enzymes" were identified that could slice chromosomes at specific locations. For the first time, this enabled with precision and reliability specific genes for specific traits to be moved from the chromosome of one kind of cell and attached to a different chromosome in a different kind of cell – even if the cells were from two different species of life. Now, imagine if a deadly gene from one virus (e.g., a trait that causes cancer or immunodeficiency) were spliced into the chromosome of an easily transmissible virus (like the one that causes the common cold) or bacterium (like the ones that line the gastrointestinal tract). The horror of this scenario, including its accidental occurrence, dampened public enthusiasm over the new biology.

To make matters worse, the horror scenario had roots in reality, even though its actual manifestation was very unrealistic. SV-40 was a virus that molecular biologists worked with as a means of delivering DNA into a eukaryotic. This virus had been isolated from monkey kidney cells in the early 1960s and had several properties that made it especially useful in laboratory experiments. It was subsequently found to be carcinogenic in hamsters, and to cause tumor-like alterations in cultured human cells. Before SV-40's carcinogenicity was identified, early batches of the polio vaccine were cultured in monkey kidney cells and later epidemiological studies showed that many of the millions of recipients of the vaccine had antibodies to the SV-40 virus (however they have not been shown to have a higher probability of developing cancer). Nevertheless, the close correlation of SV-40 with cancer led several researchers in the early 1970s to argue against using that virus – or any other toxic or carcinogenic virus – or any genetic fragment of such viruses, in recombinant DNA experiments. Adding fuel to this fire was the fact that:

> [T]he interests of most of the molecular biologists did not lie in classical bacteriology, and many had received only rudimentary instruction in handling pathogens or in the ecology of microorganisms. Any anxieties they harbored were directed more toward maintaining a competitive edge in the hunt for new paradigms, and their laboratory technique with respect to germs often reflected this priority (Frederickson, p.264).

During 1971-74, some biologists were raising concerns about the possible untoward consequences of unregulated genetic engineering experiments, while other biologists were preparing to conduct the first recombinant DNA experiments using modified SV-40 viruses and *E. coli*. All such debate and activity was occurring within the fairly small fraternity of no more than a few hundred leading molecular biologists. The situation came to a boil when Herbert Boyer of the University of California, San Francisco, "spilled the beans" at a 1973 scientific conference that he and his colleague, Stanley Cohen of Stanford University, had actually succeeded in using restriction enzymes to combine two different antibiotic-resistant plasmids and insert the hybrid genes into *E. coli*. Recall from this chapter's earlier discussion of antibiotic resistance that a virulent strain of multiply-resistant *E. coli* is an epidemiologists' nightmare. Within hours the shocked conference attendees voted to ask the National Academy of Sciences and the Institute of Medicine to convene a committee to figure out how to manage the risks of recombinant DNA research. The head of the NIH during this period described the situation as "biology approaching something akin to the nuclear physicists' chilling arrival at 'critical mass'" (Frederickson, p.271).

The Academy selected Paul Berg of Stanford University to form the requested committee. Prof. Berg was a logical choice for several reasons. Scientifically, he was at the forefront of performing recombinant DNA tricks with viruses, plasmids and *E. coli* cells, but he had voluntarily deferred doing such experiments with SV-40 based on the concerns of some scientists in the field (although he was the first to conceive of those experiments) (Rudacille, pp.217-18). Also, on his own volition, he had convened an early, albeit inconclusive, meeting (sometimes known as Asilomar I) on the subject of recombinant DNA risks. Berg formed a committee of experts in early 1974, which promptly issued a report recommending: (1) a moratorium on the experiments with the highest risk of harm, (2) strict scrutiny of any linkage of animal and non-animal DNA, (3) creation of a standing government recombinant DNA oversight group, and (4) convocation of an international meeting of the concerned scientists to discuss ways of dealing with the potential hazards of recombinant DNA molecules.

In February 1975, the recommended international meeting occurred to discuss the need for continuing the *de facto* moratorium on recombinant DNA research. The moratorium arose from a letter published in the July 24, 1974, issue of *Science* that summarized the report of Berg's committee and asked microbiologists throughout the world to voluntarily refrain from doing genetic engineering experiments until the international meeting could be convened on the subject of appropriate ways of managing the risks. The resultant meeting, now known as the Asilomar Conference (or Asilomar II), replaced the moratorium with a set of recommended isolation or containment procedures.

The Asilomar procedures varied according to a classification of risk, with obviously safe genetic experiments permitted on a benchtop, possibly dangerous experiments restricted to negative air pressure systems, and obviously dangerous ones restricted to "space suit" facilities such as Fort Detrick or Porton Down (Goodfield, pp.130-31). The recommended guidelines were ultimately adopted, in somewhat strengthened form, by the U.S. National Institutes of Health on June 23, 1976, and by other governmental agencies worldwide.

The Asilomar procedures, and their federal implementation, did not end debate over the appropriate management of recombinant DNA research. Local regulatory bodies re-argued the issues, often with more risk-averse results:

> In 1976, the controversy erupted in Cambridge, Massachusetts, when Harvard proposed to convert some rooms in the biology department into a P3 (moderately high level containment) laboratory devoted to recombinant DNA research. Scientists with offices in the building protested vehemently and took their concerns to the mayor, Alfred Velucci. In the summer of 1976, the City Council held hearings and heard testimony from those in favor of and opposed to construction of the labs, which included Nobel Prize-winning biologist George Wald and his wife and fellow biologist, Ruth Hubbard. The City Council voted on a three-month moratorium on recombinant DNA research in the city of Boston,

> a ban that would affect both Harvard and MIT, the city's premier research institutions. The council also set up a Cambridge Experimentation Review Board to draft recommendations on recombinant DNA research that were expected to be much stricter than those set by NIH after the Asilomar Conference (Rudacille, p.221).

There is no magic formula to the appropriate amount of regulation and control for a potentially hazardous activity. Different localities and countries have isolation and containment procedures that vary from those agreed to at Asilomar. The NIH itself periodically readjusts the Asilomar guidelines, although never departing from the basic structure of regulating the permissibility of research in accordance with its risk. The key point, though, is that while even potentially catastrophic risks will not block authorization of research of beneficial promise, such research is subjected to operational constraints that grow more onerous with the potential risk.

"Devil's Doctrine" Debunked

The Asilomar Conference is often pointed to as a unique example of society standing up and saying "no" to what has been called the "Devil's Doctrine" – what can be done, must be done. However, the meeting was contentious, with many if not most, of the participants dismissive of the risks of recombinant DNA, suspicious of the motives of those who wanted to restrict other scientists' research, and concerned that their scarce budgets would be wasted on expensive containment facilities. Indeed, about 10 percent of the attendees at Asilomar opposed the recommended constraints. In the words of Asilomar chronicler June Goodfield:

> Their position was and still is: no one – neither public agency nor peer group nor society – can say to a scientist, "Thou shalt not do a particular experiment" (Goodfield, p.101).

This radical position did not prevail for a number of reasons. Most of the scientists felt that their work could be accomplished within the containment constraints, and they had no strong motivation to object. Other scientists felt they had an obligation to society to minimize any possible harm from their actions, and that this obligation trumped the traditional obligation of scientists to "search for truth." Recent seeds for this latter view can be found in the aftermath of Hiroshima and Nagasaki:

> The conception of the scientist and technical person as mere spectator, a neutral bystander who observes and comments on the passing scene in ways that antiseptically avoid any involvement in it went up in the smoke of the first atomic bomb. Given the technical character of most risks that arise in a modern technologized state, there is no alternative to looking to the expert for information

> and guidance. The society, which provides for their recruitment, training, and employment, unhesitatingly expects its professional experts to adopt a certain standard of practice in which the protection of the public interest plays a central role. Such expectations form the basis of a moral obligation to apply socially fostered knowledge to society's benefit (Rescher, p.166).

But the main reason the radical position failed, and that a consensus was achieved after all, was probably due to eleventh hour presentations of the lawyer-participants. One law professor put the fear of God into the scientist-participants with his explanation of their possible legal responsibility under negligence (financial and criminal) or strict liability (regardless of whether they were at fault) for any harm caused to laboratory workers or the public.

> Listening to the lawyers predict what might happen to the decisions to be made on the morrow, the scientists stiffened their resolve to close ranks so that the world would see that the scientific community was able to finish what it had begun (Fredrickson, p.281).

Science is Neither Above the Law Nor Apart from Society

Goodfield looks at Asilomar as a turning point in scientific ethics because it marked the first time that the sciences professions formally accepted a social contract with society.

> Professional activity is not only concerned with individual rewards but with something transcendental too: whether it is improved health care or a more realistic interpretation of the law or better education for the young or, as in the case of the scientific profession, the discovery of truth. With the sole exception of the scientific profession, one other thing unites them all: services to the public are their chief object, cemented by a contractual relationship. Because of this contract the competence of a professional is appraised both internally, by his contemporaries, and externally, by the public.
>
> Accountability, in the last analysis, is the price the professions pay for their privileges. The ethical relationship that exists between society and the professions, which marks the nature of their social contract, is supported by the twin pillars of mutual responsibility and accountability to such an extent that a series of protections has grown up between both sides, designed to shield each other from malpractice or exploitation.
>
> Such an external accountability is missing from the social contract between the scientific profession and society, however, and this is the focus of the present

> dilemma. For scientists see no reason why this social contract should change, whereas society now sees every reason why it should (Goodfield, p.79).

Because genetic engineering presented a possibility of great endangerment to the public, there was no chance that scientists could any longer abstain from a social contract with society. In the words of Senator Edward Kennedy, then chairman of the U.S. Senate Committee responsible for health matters:

> It was commendable that scientists attempted to think through the social consequences of their work. It was commendable, but it was inadequate. It was inadequate because scientists alone had decided to impose the moratorium, and scientists alone had decided to lift it. Yet the factors under consideration extend far beyond their technical competence. In fact they were making public policy and they were making it in private (Goodfield, p.148).

The Asilomar Conference represented an iconic moment for a new social contract between the scientific professions and society:

> This episode of recombinant DNA could be the starting point for a new social contract both within the professions and in its external relations . . . . a contract where – as Rousseau said – each person gives up a measure of his freedom in return for the protection of freedoms for all, so as to maintain a desirable human condition (Goodfield, p.209).

Twenty-five years after Asilomar, a retrospective conference was held at the same site, and with some of the same participants. Paul Berg, the principal organizer of the first conference, noted "consensus might never have been reached if the scientists at Asilomar had not agreed to put aside the ethical issues and stick to biological hazards" (Barinaga, p.1584). However, another conference participant, Princeton University President and Chairman of the National Bioethics Advisory Commission, Harold Shapiro, emphasized Goodfield's point that "scientists owe society." Interestingly, though, of all the predictions made 25 years ago, it is the predictions of the lawyer-participants, made after dinner on the last full day of the 1975 conference, that ring most true:

> Capron then coursed across the terrain of regulation, rule making, and legislation, concluding that he hoped he had led the scientists to accept three things: some regulation is necessary, it may lead to restrictions, and public and governmental bodies would insist on having a say (Frederickson, p.281).

Asilomar leaves a twin legacy: there is a practical precedent of how to manage a new bio-threat (levels of isolation and containment), and there is an ethical precedent of how to manage a new bio-technology (open discussion along with a willingness to sacrifice scientific freedom for social security). Both of these lessons will prove to be important for xenotransplantation. Isolation and containment rules will prove to be essential for managing the risk of xenoviruses. However, of commensurate importance, xenotransplantation freedom will have to be sacrificed to satisfy global demands for the safety of public health. Furthermore, that sacrifice will only be accepted by the public – as a basis for going forward with the technology – if it is debated with the same spirit of openness (journalists and non-scientists were invited) as characterized Asilomar.

Insofar as the risk profile of xenotransplantation tracks that of recombinant DNA, the bottom line for using pig organs in man will almost surely mirror Professor Capron's bottom line for swapping DNA among life forms: some regulation is necessary, some restrictions will be enforced, and the lay public and government will have a say in what those restrictions are.

From the technologists' perspective, the good news is that society always lets promising research go forward, notwithstanding the existence of some risk of catastrophic results. On the other hand, scientists should not expect to receive a *carte blanche*, and the length of their leash will not be set solely by their peers.

Applying Asilomar to Xenotransplantation

The new social contract baptized at Asilomar resonates well with the xenotransplantation ethics debate. Here, too, there are scientific researchers who feel entitled to pursue new truths – in this case, can animal organs work in people? Allied constituencies contribute to the debate, with a clamoring for xenografts by patients and their physicians. But it is just as unreasonable to accept xenotransplantation advocates' "nothing to worry about" response to concerns regarding risks to public health as it was to accept the similar protestations on behalf of opponents to strict recombinant DNA guidelines.

> Hubris is the constant threat. No idea is more intoxicating than the one that we can take control of the processes of life. Scientists are human beings. Like the rest of us, they are prone to overambition. The problem is that, precisely because of the effectiveness of science, their mistakes tend to be catastrophic (Appleyard, p.17).

The antidote developed at Asilomar to "scientific overambition" is that a double-defense of isolation and containment provides adequate protection against the hubris of biotechnology:

- *Isolate* anything thought to be harmful from the environment where it can cause harm (e.g., outside a laboratory);

- *Contain* anything that might be harmful in a way that gives it only a remote chance of surviving where it could cause harm (e.g., outside of the laboratory environment).

Applying these guidelines to xenotransplantation would teach us to:

- *Isolate* xenograft animals from anything thought to be harmful to the human environment, such as known viruses, harmful bacteria and other pathogens (e.g., xenograft herds must be from specified pathogen free sources);
- *Contain* any xenograft that might be harmful so that it has only a remote chance of transmission into society (e.g., don't permit xenograft recipients to donate blood).

Recalling that endangerment of public health means more people may be hurt than helped by a medical technology, it is only logical to isolate the risk in expanding zones of containment so that any harm is nipped in the bud – at least until it is known that xenotransplantation clearly comes down on the helpful side of this endangerment equation. In this way, the numbers of people who may be endangered will never become too great as compared to the number of people who are helped with xenografts. Practically, this means that the risks of xenotransplantation need to be ranked, and an appropriate level of containment needs to be associated with each rank. For example:

- a person known to be infected with a transmissible xenogeneic virus should be isolated in quarantine (at least until more is known), whereas a person who might be infected with a transmissible xenogeneic virus could be contained by prohibition of blood donation;
- porcine organs that are known to be pathogen-free should be transplantable with minimum restrictions, whereas porcine organs that may harbor pathogens should be restricted to laboratories;
- bio-monitoring for xenogeneic viruses can be thought of as a form of spatio-temporal containment, pursuant to which xenograft recipients submit to comprehensive lab tests in the first year after xenotransplantation, moderate lab tests during the next couple of years, and modest lab tests annually thereafter.

The World Health Organization has, in fact, adopted a containment philosophy for xenotransplantation in their 1998 Guidance on Infectious Disease Prevention and Management document:

> Recipient follow-up is a precautionary measure for containing infectious agents and preventing their spread to the general population. Any containment steps undertaken, however, must be proportionate to the risk of dissemination into the general population assigned to the particular agent of interest.
>
> When implemented, containment steps should be initiated immediately, and continued until a determination is made that there is no further risk to the general population. These steps may require quarantine or other physical restrictions on the individual recipient. Adopted procedures should be periodically reevaluated to assure applicability and appropriateness (WHO 1998, p.13).

The Precautionary Principle

Asilomar is a "risk-based" approach to regulation that may be contradistinguished from what is increasingly called the "precautionary" approach (Appell, p.18). Both approaches are somewhat schizophrenically combined in the newly adopted Cartagena Biosafety Protocol (a successor to the 1992 Rio Declaration on the Environment and Development), which regulates the transborder shipment of non-pharmaceutical genetically modified living organisms (such as GM food and seed) (*Decision*, 20). The precautionary approach dictates that biotechnology may be deemed unsafe by a country until proven safe (UNEP, p.47; Appell, p.19), and regulators may use that argument to block the importation of a product (Miller and Conko, p.360). On the other hand, the risk-based approach is adopted by the Protocol as a guide for national risk assessments and it, like Asilomar, "focuses on the biological characteristics of the individual products" and "depends on the stratification of organisms into risk categories according to the consensus judgments of independent scientific experts" (Miller and Conko, p.360).

The Cartagena Biosafety Protocol is evidence that the world, in general, is ready to accept the risks of introducing recombinant into the global environment DNA living organisms. In this sense, the Cartagena Biosafety Protocol represents an elevation of the Asilomar process to the broadest international level. Oppositely, the world is not yet ready to permit biotechnology to trump national sovereignty *de jure* – and thus individual countries can still block biotechnology imports by playing the "precautionary" card. Left unmentioned is the *de facto* trumping of national sovereignty that biotechnology accomplishes by virtue of the extraordinary mobility of microbes in the closed ecosystem of earth.

Were the Protocol or an extrapolation of it applied to xenograft recipients, the analogous rules would be that (a) a xenograft recipient would need a special visa before visiting a country for the first time, (b) the Biosafety Clearing House would be consulted as to whether the recipient's xenograft was of a class known to cause any biosafety hazards, and (c) notwithstanding a "clean bill of health" from a risk assessment standpoint on the recipient's xenograft, the destination country could still deny him a visa as a "precaution." WHO opined that the principle of precaution should be applied to xenotransplantation, although it does not require "a total absence of risk" ("Emerging," para. 4.3). National sovereignty wins *de jure*, but if the xenograft recipient is spreading a virus, national sovereignty will *de facto* lose. Consequently, in the microbial arena, it is in everyone's best interest for everyone to be part of the risk management game.

A criticism of the Asilomar regime is that it may fail to take into account unanticipated harmful consequences of seemingly harmless actions. For example, medicines have been approved based on safety in thousands of volunteers, but have then been withdrawn when harmful side effects manifested themselves years later. Barry Commoner is famous for his First Law of Ecology: "Everything is Connected to Everything Else" (Commoner, "The Closing," p.46). He argues that "a small perturbation in one place may have large, distant, long-delayed effects," and "any major man-made change in a natural system is likely to be detrimental to that system" (Commoner, "The Closing," pp.39-41). Consequently, notwithstanding all of the Asilomar-type "isolation and containment" that will be applied to xenotransplantation, it is still inevitable, in a Commoner view, that adverse effects will materialize in the bio-environment:

> [C]onfidence is based on the false premise that it is as safe to shuffle genes in the world as it is in the lab. We do not know that because we know very little about the complex interactions of genes and the proteins for which they provide the blueprints (Appleyard, p.17).

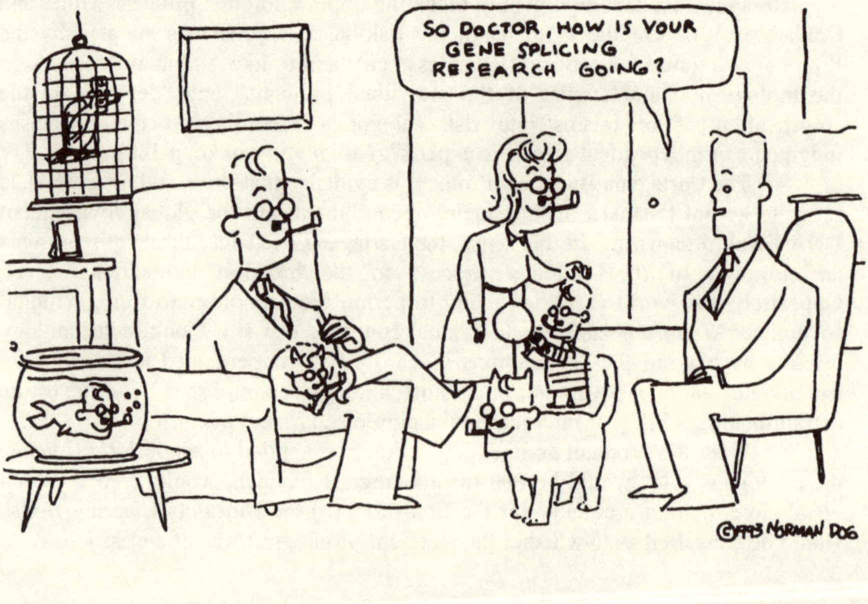
SO DOCTOR, HOW IS YOUR GENE SPLICING RESEARCH GOING?
©1993 NORMAN DOG

However, it can be fairly argued, that xenotransplantation is a scientific achievement that is proceeding in full consonance with Commoner-type principles. First, discussions of ethics have been in the forefront, even buttressed by moratoria, not quashed by the military or corporate secrecy that Commoner so disdains (Commoner, pp.16-22). Second, there is a robust appreciation of the possible effects of xenotransplantation on the human environment. Consequently, it is generally agreed that Asilomar-type isolation and containment procedures must be a *sine qua non* of xenotransplantation; indeed, as described in chapter III, procedures of that sort are already required by the FDA and the XIRA. Finally, it is understood that ultimately there is a price to pay for "fooling Mother Nature" with xenografts in immunocompromised bodies. That price is vigilant surveillance, monitoring and control of emerging zoonoses. Chapter VII provides a detailed framework for the funding and implementation of such a xenozoonosis surveillance network.

It must be recognized that the Asilomar regime has not forestalled strong public opposition to one of recombinant DNA's harvests – genetically modified (GM) foods. This opposition exists notwithstanding the lack of proven harm from such foods and their development, pursuant to Asilomar guidelines. Public opposition, therefore, may be based on perceived non-measurable harm, or even on ideological objections.

The response of the Asilomar regime to such objections is that risk containment is not a guarantee of safety. Recombinant DNA guidelines are meant to strike an optimum balance between technological progress and public safety; to reflect the responsibility of the scientific community to the society that makes their research possible. Even eliminating Reschler Rule III risks, those of "effective zero probability," still results in "stultification." Nevertheless, levels of risk containment are certainly not a talisman against adverse public opinion. And the tendency of public opinion is to overestimate the probability of remote risks and to underestimate the probability of likely risks.

In summary, xenotransplantation can be risk-managed with the understanding that it provides antibiotic-like health benefits but is susceptible to Asilomar-type regulation and control. The "realistic scenario is that, perhaps, one in 1000 xenograft recipients may pick up a porcine retrovirus and, if detected, that infection may be treatable by anti-retroviral therapy and would not spread to the patient's contacts" (Weiss et al., p.24). However, it is also true that a "worst case scenario would be a major new viral pandemic like HIV/AIDS" (Weiss et al., p.24). Consequently, the detection and treatment of xenograft-borne viruses, and the regulation and control of xenotransplantation, cannot reasonably be affairs left to the initiative of individual countries. A global plan must be contemplated from the start.

Asilomar-Type Rules and Antibiotic-Type Risks on a Global Stage

This chapter commenced with the observation that while a compelling case can be made for a right to xenotransplantation, that right is not absolute. It cannot trump the interests of the collective in avoiding undue endangerment of public health. The body of this chapter showed, through comparison with precedents such as antibiotic drug and recombinant DNA technology, that the mere risk of xenogeneic disease is not a sufficient basis of collective concern to quash xenotransplantation. To the contrary, because the acceptability of risks are perceived in relation to the importance of the rewards for which the risks are undertaken, the collective is likely to be receptive to the risks of xenotransplantation. Indeed, the death toll from technology itself constitutes some 20 percent of all mortality (Rescher, p.183). Technology is of obvious importance to the collective, and, as discussed in chapter V, the need for human health is paramount.

The public health endangerment potential of xenotransplantation is roughly analogous to that posed by liberal use of antibiotics. Society accepts the latter, notwithstanding thousands of deaths and billions of dollars worth of morbidity, because great importance is attached to increasing the health of sick members of the collective. Society is, therefore, also likely to accept xenotransplantation because it, too, addresses – perhaps even more vitally – the all-important basic human need for health. On the other hand, society is wiser for its 20th century experiences with unleashed technologies – from antibiotics and atomic energy to recombinant DNA and industrial pollution. Consequently, it is reasonable for society to endeavor to apply its wisdom to minimize the risks of xenotransplantation, a step taken only haltingly, belatedly and incompletely, with antibiotics. The Asilomar experience provides the template for xenotransplantation risk reduction: isolation and containment.

A Little Bit of Risk is Not a Bad Thing

Is xenotransplantation worth the risk? The answer appears to be yes because by "worth the risk" it is meant: does the procedure unduly endanger public health? Xenotransplantation is unlikely to endanger public health any more than antibiotics. How does one know that xenotransplantation's adverse effects will be limited? Because public policy demands, as part of the social compact with the sciences epitomized by the Asilomar Conference, that reasonable controls on biotechnology development are the *quid pro quo* of societal support for the science. Reasonable controls on xenotransplantation, like those on recombinant DNA work, ensure, to the extent practical, via risk-adjusted isolation and containment procedures, that adverse effects will be discovered before much harm is caused. Consequently, it can be expected that the benefits to public health from xenotransplantation will far exceed any harm it inflicts. For these reasons, xenotransplantation is worth the risk – especially so given the all-important goal of optimum human health that it promises to deliver to millions suffering from end-stage organ failure.

The promise of xenotransplantation stands on the twin pillars of health enhancement (there is a right) and risk management (terms of society accepting the obligation). Each of these pillars are relatively solid in Western countries due to their national wealth and advanced public health infrastructure. With such an infrastructure, clinical trials can be rigorous, pathogen-free source pigs can be monitored, xenotransplantation operations will be paid for and xenograft patient infection risks will be contained. Unfortunately, the same cannot be said of the public health infrastructure elsewhere in the world. How can the promise of xenotransplantation be shared with the developing world?

Excessively risky procedures outside the West will create a xenogeneic epidemic risk worldwide. Be that as it may, when the West decides to assume the risks of xenotransplantation because of the importance of saving lives, it is putting the rest of the world at risk as well – without countervailing benefits. Because viruses "need no passports" the conflict between public and private interests in xenotransplantation cannot be resolved solely on a national level. Xenotransplantation, like antibiotics and recombinant DNA, poses global dilemmas. Consequently, the debate goes beyond bioethics; a *geo*ethical solution is needed as well.

The need for a comprehensive new "geoethical" solution with the advent of xenotransplantation may be looked at as an example of the Daedalus effect in science (Blumberg and Fox, p.390). The mythical Daedalus was like a super-engineer, always developing new and clever technological solutions to ancient problems. Each of his solutions, however, inevitably gave rise to joy as well as sorrow. He looked at the sorrow opportunistically, seeing in it the seeds of another solution. So it is with science generally: the advent of antibiotics has resulted in resistance; the advent of recombinant DNA research has resulted in *a priori* legal restrictions. It should be expected that as a scientific solution to unnecessary death, xenotransplantation will have a Daedalus effect. With proper foresight and preemptive action, that effect can be one of a regulatory regime, such as Daedalus' respect of an altitude limit for flying with wings of wax, or as with recombinant DNA's legal regime of isolation and containment levels. Science that is blinded to the Daedalus effect all too often ends up mired in reckless consequences, as happened when Daedalus' son, Icarus, ignored the altitude rules, or as would be the case with unregulated xenotransplantation.

Risk Bearers of the World, Unite!

In fact, xenogeneic viruses exemplify a class of risks born of industrial success that typically transcend national borders. Ulrich Beck is widely recognized for his thesis that modernization carries with it a transformation of society from one that is nationalist, labor-class oriented and concerned with the distribution of wealth to one that is globalist, issue-oriented and concerned with the distribution of risk (Beck, p.20). He notes that hazardous side effects are the pollution of wealth creation. Applied to xenotransplantation, Beck's thesis would state that in the quest for greater health via organ replacement, it must be expected that there will be side effects of potential xenogeneic diseases.

Beck's theory would then imply that very soon the concern over distribution of the risks of such diseases will at least equal, and perhaps overshadow, concerns over fair access to the lifesaving transplantation procedures:

> In this sense, the risk society produces new antagonisms of interest and a new type of community of the endangered whose political carrying capacity remains, however, an open question. To the extent to which modernization hazards generalize and thus abolish the remaining zones of non-involvement, the risk society (in contrast to class society) develops a tendency to unify the victims in global risk positions. In the limiting case, then, friend and foe, east and west, above and below, city and country, south and north are all exposed to the leveling pressure of the exponentially increasing risks of civilization. Risk societies are not class societies – that is not saying enough. They contain within themselves a grass-roots developmental dynamics that destroys boundaries, through which the people are forced together in the uniform position of civilization's self-endangering.
>
> The potential for self-endangering developed by civilization in the modernization process thus also makes the utopia of a world society a little more real or at least more urgent. People in the nineteenth century had to learn, on penalty of economic ruin, to subject themselves to the conditions of industrial society and wage labor. In just the same way, they also have to learn today as in the future, under the shadow of an apocalypse of civilization, to sit down at a table to find and enforce solutions to the self-inflicted endangering that crosses all borders (Beck, pp.47-48).

It is to these solutions of global "self-inflicted endangering" that this book now turns. These solutions must be of a geoethical nature, for the body being treated with xenotransplantation is not just the one on the surgeon's table, but also the body politic spread across the globe. This geographically diffuse and altogether unwitting "patient" will feel the side effects of risk just as assuredly as does the prostate patient gain the reward of renewed life. Consequently, if mankind wants to grasp the fruit of longer life, then it must adjust itself to Beck's reality of a "world society" – in this case one in which global healthcare is not utopia, but an urgent and indispensable solution waiting for practical and vigilant enforcement.

Conclusion

In a sound byte, xenotransplantation in the U.S. and Europe creates a risk of unleashing an AIDS-type epidemic on the world. The human species is enough of a risk-taker that not even that large a potential catastrophe blackballs a promising technology such as xenotransplantation. However, basic human decency requires one to ask a neighbor's permission before doing something that risks blowing up his house. In exactly the same vein – with our eyes wide open to the fact that developing countries face untold millions of deaths from AIDS while the U.S. and Europe keep most of their HIV+ patients alive with expensive drugs – basic human decency requires the risk-makers in the North to seek the approval of the risk-bearers in the South before creating a catastrophic risk.

As Commoner prophesied some 50 years ago:

> Every major advance in the technological competence of man has enforced revolutionary changes in the economic and political structure of society. The present age of technology is no exception to this rule of history. We already known the enormous benefits it can bestow; we have begun to perceive its frightful threats. The political crisis generated by this knowledge is upon us. Science can reveal the depth of this crisis, but only social action can resolve it. Science can now serve society by exposing the crisis of modern technology to the judgment of all mankind. Only this judgment can determine whether the knowledge that science has given us shall destroy humanity or advance the welfare of man (Commoner, p.132).

In the war against disease, to use H.H. Frost's maxim, "every mistake is excusable except inactivity and refusal to take risks." And, as Harris reminds us, it "would surely be negligent to deny human beings the benefits and protections of new technology one moment longer than is necessary" (Harris, "The Ethics," p.324). However, when the risk is shifted to a global population of innocents, Commoner's plea for "judgment" is also a call for the global healthcare of a world society – as revolutionary a change as that is. Applying the Asilomar lessons of isolation and containment to xenoviruses requires nothing less than at least a basic, surveillance-competent, global health care system. The right to health care may demand more, and Beck's world society may demand more. But from a risk management standpoint, some kind of a global health care system is an inevitable, minimum concomitant of xenotransplantation.

Chapter VII

A Geoethical Solution to the Conflict Between Private and Public Interests in Xenotransplantation

The preceding chapters demonstrate that logical extensions of existing precedent support a right to xenotransplantation. Underlying the right is an outstanding need for xenografts to help save the lives of millions of people, and the compelling basic human need for health care. The right to xenotransplantation is constrained in three key ways: (1) respect for animals, (2) budget, and (3) public health concerns.

This book has shown that, at least in theory, each of the three constraints on access to xenotransplantation can be adequately addressed. Appropriate animal care regulations can offer pigs appropriate levels of respect. Transparent health care budgeting procedures can implement xenograft rationing fairly. Biosurveillance can be conducted consistently with the human rights of the patients.

Introduction

Availability of the preconditions for xenotransplantation in theory does not imply their implementation in practice. What happens to the right to xenotransplantation when its concomitant constraints fail to be realized? What happens to the right when one of its preconditions never congeals in one or more countries, while other countries scrupulously observe the rules? What happens if one or more countries unilaterally decide to use non-SPF-free pigs for xenografts, or if word leaks out that their pigs spend their entire lives hooked to medical tubing in a sterile box? The world is affected, either by being placed at heightened disease risk (non-SPF-pigs) or by having its conscience shocked (boxing the pigs for life). Who suffers if one or more countries decide to forego lifelong biosurveillance of xenograft recipients? The world suffers because it is placed at an unnecessarily higher risk of xenozoonotic individuals unwittingly spreading a new disease worldwide.

Logically, the right to xenotransplantation should not be implemented anywhere its preconditions are not present. The logic behind the requirement of *universal* compliance with public health constraints is that viruses don't respect borders. Reckless xenotransplantation in one country places the entire world at risk of pandemic disease. *Consequently, if at least a basic global public health capability cannot be put in place as part and parcel of clinical xenotransplantation, then xenotechnology should not go forward.* To do otherwise would be seeking a "free lunch" in man's interference with xenobiology. Chapter VI made quite clear that those "free lunches" are illusory. Nature extracts payment for interference, and no country in the world can afford another AIDS-type pandemic.

The foregoing course of reasoning must also consider the momentum of human affairs. Once xenotransplantation is set in motion, the neglect of preconditions in one country is unlikely to cause an abandonment of the procedure in other countries (or even in the lax country). The clamor of a growing xenotransplantation constituency – doctors, hospitals, patients, families, friends – will be too strong. But such an eventuality imposes unacceptable risk upon the entire world community. Consequently, practical realization of the right to xenotransplantation requires a *mandatory* global public health enforcement regime. *If this regime cannot be brought into being, then xenotransplantation should not be brought into being.*

This chapter will first address the philosophical underpinnings of a new global enforcement organization for xenobiology (GEOX) – a mandatory implementation of Asilomar-type isolation and containment procedures in the context of public health and xenotransplantation. These philosophical considerations contemplate the elevation of bioethics to *geoethics*, and hence introduce a new interplay between individualism and communitarianism, between rights-based and community-based approaches to health care ethics.

The chapter will then conclude with a practical implementation of the GEOX concept, including its substantive elements, its finances and a legal pathway for its realization. GEOX cannot be realized without global participation in the development of the regime. As shown in chapter VI for non-pharmaceutical GM organisms, countries will not blindly cede public health authority to an international regime. They must have an opportunity to understand why it is in their interest to do so, and to explain how their unique circumstances should be best accommodated. Like democracy on a global scale, participation of the governed is the best assurance of the support of the governed.

In essence, the practical implementation of GEOX recapitulates its philosophical foundation as a necessarily global communitarian accommodation of an individual's right to optimal health care. That right to health care is, itself, born of society's need to ensure that its own members can fulfill their roles. Consequently, the conflict between private rights and public interests in xenotransplantation is resolved by recognizing that every national society owes a risk management duty to the world. This global duty, executable via GEOX, arises in exchange for the world permitting national health care duties to be discharged to individuals via the inherently risky technology of xenotransplantation.

Bioethics has guided the application of medical technology to individuals with a set of norms based around autonomy (individuals must be respected as individuals), nonmalfeasance (avoid causing harm to individuals) and beneficence (only do what is expected to benefit an individual) (R. Fox, p.237). When medical technology has global impact, as does xenotransplantation, the individual-focused norms of bioethics must be trumped by a new set of world-focused norms. This might be called *geoethics*.

A pair of concepts similar to the bioethics-geoethics dialectic are microethics and macroethics:

> General ethical principles may be applied at individual and community levels. At the level of the individual (microethics), ethics governs how one person should relate to another and the moral claims of each member of a community. At the level of the community, ethics applies to how one community relates to another, and to how a community treats each of its members (including prospective members) and members of other groups with different cultural values (macroethics). Procedures that are unethical at one level cannot be justified merely because they are considered ethically acceptable at the other (CIOMS, p.11).

In a similar vein, just as a doctor should not *bioethically* experiment on a patient without their informed consent, a country should not *geoethically* experiment on humanity, via introduction of xenogeneic viruses into the human blood pool, without its consent. However, the bioethically *appropriate* consent of an individual to be a xenograft recipient does *not* justify the geoethically *in*appropriate endangerment of the human race. Unethical procedures at a global level cannot be justified simply because they are ethical at an individual level.

The content of geoethically acceptable social policies can only be elucidated via discourse among all participants. However, the centerpiece is no longer "how do I treat this person?" The mission statement must now be "how do we manage the global risks of a procedure than can add life to millions of people?" Because the "patient" is now a community and not a person, the norms must also be more geoethical than bioethical. The norms of bioethics remain important on the microscopic scale. They will, however, need now to operate within a macroscopic universe governed by a new set of geoethical rules. Generally speaking, those geoethical rules provide:

I. Conduct only those activities of potential global effect that promote the greatest relative fulfillment of basic human needs in the most distressed parts of the world (Benefit Principle);

II. Implement activities of potential global effect only in such manner as achieves the consent of all parties who may be adversely affected by such activities, through their representatives (Risk Principle);

III. Activities of potential global effect must self-finance the means and methods of independent assurance of their compliance with global norms (Assurance Principle).

Once an activity complies with the foregoing geoethical principles on a macroscopic level, traditional bioethical principles of beneficence, non-malfeasance and autonomy can apply microscopically, to individual patients and their health care providers.

Practical Implementation of Geoethical Xenotransplantation

A monologic book, of course, is no substitute for discursive argumentation among all the stakeholders in xenotransplantation. Nevertheless, by engaging in a certain amount of "role playing" it is possible to set forth likely outcomes of such discussions. These likely outcomes can serve at least two useful roles. First, their practicality (or impracticality) serves to validate (or invalidate) the resolutions proposed in this book of the conflict between private and public interests in xenotransplantation. Second, the likely outcomes can serve as "strawmen" frameworks for real world discussions of xenotransplantation policy.

As described above, a GEOX is needed to resolve the conflict between private and public interests in xenotransplantation. Hence, proposed structures for the global enforcement organization will be set forth as the substantive element of the proposed xenotransplantation policy. The text will next explore the feasibility of financing GEOX with fees earned from xenotransplantation procedures. Finally, probable legal pathways will be described through which discourse can occur and become reified in mandatory norms.

Who Will Do What To Whom?

When participants get together to discuss xenotransplantation policies they will focus on the issue that gives rise to mandatory global enforcement requirements – the need for Asilomar-type rules and regulations that can contain and isolate any xenogeneic disease risk. The range of possible activities of such an enforcement organization, though, will be quite broad:

"Minimal Competence"

- Certify pathogen-free acceptability of donor animals;
- Certify compliance with xenograft recipient monitoring rules;
- Certify compliance with xenogeneic disease quarantine rules.

"Maximal Competence" (includes Minimal Competence set as well)

- Determine ethical acceptability standards for donor animals;
- Ensure equitable global participation in xenograft recipient pool;
- Conduct public health-based global surveillance for emerging bio-threats.

It would be a fairly straightforward matter for a group of largely Western experts to get together, perhaps via an industry group such as the *Transplantation Society* (www.transplantation-soc.org), and decide to offer the Minimal Competence certifications outlined above. Alternatively, the regulatory body of a Western country, such as the FDA or the UK's Xenotransplantation Interim Regulatory Authority (UKXIRA), can solicit input from local experts and promulgate donor herd, xenograft monitoring, and xenogeneic disease quarantine rules and procedures.

Problems with Minimal Competence Regimes

Both the United Kingdom and the United States normative guidelines are Minimal Competence measures that do not represent an adequate *moral response* to the conflict between private and public interests in xenotransplantation. The reason for this shortcoming is that none of these measures were developed pursuant to an ethical discourse among all the parties to whom xenotransplantation risk will be distributed.

The risks of xenotransplantation are necessarily allocated worldwide. Consequently, notwithstanding the considerable expertise of the FDA or XIRA, worldwide entities have a moral right to participate in the extrapolation of the norms that affect them. The risks of xenotransplantation are also necessarily allocated across all sectors of society. Consequently, even a global body of experts such as the *Transplantation Society* cannot morally exclude laypeople from the promulgation of certification procedures and standards.

Now, a truly participatory set of discussions could, in theory, result in a set of xenotransplantation norms that track the Minimal Competence rules set forth above. In practice, this is unlikely. Some parties will inevitably ask, "what benefit is there for me to accept these risks, which the certification procedures admittedly reduce but do not eliminate?" Others may ask, "does our financial inability to monitor public health preclude us from the benefits of xenotransplantation, but not from the risks of xenogeneic disease?" Yet other parties may express concern that life scientists are capable of defining pathogen free conditions for xenografts, but lack the training to specify ethical standards for raising and sacrificing the donor herds, as described in chapter IV's discussion of harm to animals.

If the Minimal Competence rules won't achieve agreement from all the parties affected by xenotransplantation, how much further must they be expanded to achieve such agreement? In the first instance, rules that militate against developing country participation in the fruits of xenotransplantation (strict requirements for specified pathogen free herds and expensive infection control requirements in hospitals) are very likely to give rise to demands that developing country citizens at least have a reasonable chance to access Western xenotransplantation operation centers. In addition, xenotransplantation rules that mandate surveillance of all populations for emerging zoonoses are likely to fuel demands for actual health care to those populations within developing countries. It will likely be argued that a country that cannot afford to provide basic health care to a population cannot afford to take blood samples from them. Public health interests will also advocate for the new paradigm that health care is an obligation of epidemiological surveillance (CIOMS, p.15).

A demand for some measure of global health care will also arise from claims that it is simply too unjust – even flagrantly so, in a conscience-shocking sense – to ask developing countries to participate in a legal regime that vectors billions of dollars into extending industrialized life expectancy beyond seven decades while their own populations die prematurely for want of basic health services. Considering these claims, if one was to predict what it would take to get universal agreement to a xenotransplantation treaty that minimizes the risks of xenogeneic diseases, it would very likely be something quite similar to the set of norms labeled above as "Maximal Competence." These norms address the claims of those to whom the xenorisks are disproportionately allocated – developing countries lacking advanced health care systems – with an allotment of Western xenotransplantation procedures for their citizenry in need of the same (subject to fair waiting lists rules), and with the frank provision of basic health care services in seriously underserved areas.

Maximal Competence Regime is More Realistic

Examining the Maximal Competence set of norms, every participant in the global discussion (e.g., even very poor countries) could see here a benefit (e.g., minimal health care services as part of disease surveillance) worth incurring the risks of xenotransplantation. At the same time, those who benefit most directly from xenotransplantation (e.g., Western countries) would also see a logical nexus with the additional benefits (e.g., health care surveillance for emerging infectious diseases) sought by others. In addition, even permitting access to something like 10 percent of xenotransplantation operations in the West for developing country residents is justifiable: "the prevention of renegade experiments in the developing world is as much enlightened self-interest as benevolent regard for our fellow residents on this planet" (Chapman, p.70).

A GEOX that operated pursuant to the Maximal Competence norms would need to be staffed and financed to carry out the following activities:

1. *Certify that porcine organs used in xenografts are from specified pathogen-free herds that are raised and sacrificed in an ethical manner.* This would require promulgating the necessary breeding rules that must

be met, inspecting the herds to ensure compliance with the rules, and making sure that transplant centers use only those xenografts that are certified by GEOX.

2. *Require that acceptance criteria for xenograft programs are globally inclusive and based on informed consent adequate to cover post-operative monitoring and quarantine, if necessary.* This would require promulgating the necessary medical center xenograft program rules that must be met, auditing the programs to ensure compliance with the rules, and making sure that xenotransplantation is performed only at centers that are so certified by GEOX.

    a. Program rules that ensure global inclusiveness should provide, for example, that 5-10 percent of the xenograft procedures will be allotted for patients from countries with no xenograft programs, on a first-come, first-served medical need basis, subject to priority for patients from countries that have not yet benefited from a xenograft from that medical center.

    b. Informed consent program rules would have to include a novel provision that consent to lifelong biosample monitoring and, if need be, quarantine and/or prohibition of exchanging bodily fluids, could not be later withdrawn.

    c. In order to ensure enforcement of these rules, the patients may also need to agree to waive aspects of their medical confidentiality rights.

3. *Conduct in-country surveillance for incipient signs of new zoonotic disease via national monitoring programs, or if adequate, new health care stations.* This will require promulgating the details of an adequate global surveillance program for emerging infectious disease threats, implementing this program via national health services where possible, and actually constructing minimal national health service stations where necessary to achieve the objectives of the program.

    a. It may be very difficult to determine whether an emerging infectious disease threat is xenozoonotic or just zoonotic in origin, and hence it is logical (and efficient) for the global surveillance program to search for signs of any new disease.

    b. In countries with working national health services, the surveillance program can be accomplished via rules that require random testing for new pathogens of blood samples taken for other purposes, during routine or emergency doctor visits.

    c. In countries without working health services, it will be necessary to establish a network of medical stations that the local population feels comfortable visiting for basic health care needs, and, in exchange, consents to random biosample monitoring for new pathogens.

Point 3c above is a revolutionary requirement. It is tantamount to tasking GEOX with the creation of a global basic health care capability, albeit only in places where such capability is currently lacking. However, it is fully consistent with current world health policy, since WHO recognizes that in "many parts of the world health systems are ill-equipped to cope with present demands," and governments should "diversify the sources of service provision" (WHO 1999, p.xi). For the one billion people in the world who lack basic health care, this revolution will likely make a dramatic difference in their quality of life – "the World Bank has estimated that a lack of essential clinical services is responsible for between 11 and 24 percent of the global burden of disease" (Mann, p.441). And, consistent with the Benefit Principle, while xenotransplantation is an inequality in favor of Western countries, by implementing xenotransplantation via GEOX the greatest benefits will inure to the least advantaged members of society, those without any health care at all.

Not Pie in the Sky

While the foregoing list of tasks for GEOX appear to be substantial, they are not beyond the scope of a world organization, and nor do they rise to the lofty realm of a utopian dream. To the contrary, analogous tasks are carried out today by other international organizations. And the hallmarks of utopia – perfect social harmony and equality of a society's members – are nowhere in evidence (Touraine, p.19). Before, during and after the creation of GEOX there will be gross inequality of access to xenotransplantation. The rich will still get more organs and live longer, due to a very imperfect process of obtaining the consent of the poor in exchange for a niggardly granting of concessions, such as basic health care.

Numerous legal treaties detail certification-type procedures and operational rules for all manner of global activities. The International Civil Aviation Organization (ICAO), the World Health Organization (WHO), the International Atomic Energy Agency (IAEA) and the International Telecommunication Union (ITU) are just a few of the many global organizations with responsibilities analogous to those set forth above for GEOX. In addition, the domain of microbe management is also well within the scope of international treaties.

On January 24, 2000, most of the world's countries (but not the U.S.) adopted the "Cartagena Protocol on Biosafety to the Convention on Biological Diversity." This document provides an Asilomar-like regulatory regime for "any living organism that possesses a novel combination of genetic material obtained through the use of modern biotechnology" in transboundary movement, other than pharmaceuticals for humans. In particular, no genetically modified organism may be shipped to another country except pursuant to a well-documented risk assessment and risk management procedure, which the Protocol specifies in detail. In addition, the risk assessment and management report must be favorably reviewed by an internationally-staffed Biosafety Clearing-House and accepted by the receiving country (UNEP, pp.44-65).

It is perhaps only in those areas most intrusive upon national sovereignty – mandatory allotments for non-citizens to participate in xenograft programs, and actual establishment of national health care stations under international control – that GEOX ventures furthest beyond the current envelope of global organizational competence. However, if such intrusions result from consensus among all the affected parties, then there is obviously no objection to them. On the other hand, if the argumentative discourse over risk management determines that such measures are not necessary, then this far-reaching aspect of GEOX is a non-issue.

It may reasonably be asked if the global public health surveillance prong of GEOX is not a bit of "overkill" in the management of xenozoonotic infections, especially since it carries with it a purported need to establish health care stations throughout the developing world. However, a principal recommendation of all groups grappling with the antibiotic resistance problem described at length in chapter VI, and other emerging diseases, is to establish a global public health surveillance network.[1] The American Society for Microbiology Task Force on Antibiotic Resistance concluded there "is an urgent need for effective domestic and global surveillance of antibiotic resistance in animals and humans." The Institute of Medicine concluded its 1998 study of the problem with a clear note of alarm:

> No country in the world today has a reliable, longitudinal, full-service antimicrobial resistance surveillance program . . . . Redressing these deficits is crucial in global and national public health terms, and the most powerful case possible must be made for urgent and substantial response (Institute of Medicine 1998, p.24).

---

[1] In fact, a number of international surveillance systems exist but they are limited to particular diseases and, in most cases, subsets of countries. These existing systems include Centro de Epidemiologia Molecular/Network for Epidemiologic Tracking of Antibiotic-Resistant Pathogens (CEM/NET), WHO Collaborating Center for International Monitoring of Bacterial Resistance to Antimicrobial Agents (supported by the Pharmaceutical Research and Manufacturers of America and the International Society of Infectious Diseases), WHO Gonococcal Antimicrobial Surveillance Programme, SENTRY (supported by Bristol-Myers Squibb), DoD Global Emerging Infections Surveillance and Response System (supported by the U.S. Department of Defense), Antibiotic Resistance and Emerging Susceptibility Patterns in Europe (ARTEMIS), Eurosurveillance, Salm-Net, The Alexander Project (supported by SmithKline Beecham), and Infectious Disease Early Warning System. Many other national surveillance systems exist as well.

Dr. William Foege, a former director of the Centers for Disease Control in Atlanta, has also advocated for a global surveillance program. His view is that "international and domestic American health were so thoroughly integrated by the 1990s due to globalization of the microbes that it was impossible to ensure a disease-free existence for people in North America and Western Europe without providing similar assurances for residents of Azerbaijan, Cote d'Ivoire, and Bangladesh" (Garrett, p.609).

Simply put, without global public health surveillance, it will be impossible to implement xenotransplantation consistently with the Asilomar principles of isolation and containment because it may not be known if a dangerous virus escaped until it is too widespread to contain. And there do not appear to be any "insurmountable legal obstacles" to such a surveillance program (Davis, p.46). However, because the "quality of a surveillance system is only as good as the quality of the data collected," it is crucial that the people under surveillance agree to participate:

> Acceptability reflects the willingness of individuals and organizations to participate in the system. The acceptability of a system depends on the perceived public health importance of the event under surveillance, the recognition of the contribution of individuals to the system, and how much time is needed to make the reports. The surveillance method must be acceptable not only to the collectors of the data, but also to the subjects (Declich and Canter, pp.293, 297).

While there are many ways to obtain public health surveillance information over time, the advantage of doing so in conjunction with the provision of routine health care is that any health problems uncovered can promptly be therapeutically addressed. Indeed, the evolving concept of public health surveillance includes responsibility to follow-up on findings.

> During the past 20 years the concept of surveillance was expanded further. At the 1968 World Health Assembly Technical Discussions, surveillance was said to imply the responsibility of following up to see that effective action had been taken . . . . The 1986 CDC definition of surveillance . . . states that the final link in the surveillance chain is the application of these data to prevention and control (Declich and Canter, p.287).

In the case of xenogeneic viruses, a logical surveillance program would call for a blood sample to be drawn from all surveillance stations for routine testing for known and unknown viruses at a centralized location. The incentive for people to agree to this sampling would be the provision to them of emergency or basic health station services (Otten, p.245). Such incentivization is not in lieu of informed consent, which should still be required for any bio-surveillance information that can be linked back to an individual.

The Council for International Organizations of the Medical Sciences (CIOMS) recommended in 1991 that, preferably, names be deleted in such surveillance studies to preserve confidence (Hahn, p.185). Unfortunately, this level of anonymity can interfere with therapeutic follow-up. Fortunately the CIOMS Guidelines for epidemiological studies also permit:

> *Linked information*, which may be:
>
> - anonymous, when the information cannot be linked to the person to whom it refers except by a code or other means known only to that person, and the investigator cannot know the identity of the person;
> - non-nominal, when the information can be linked to the person by a code (not including personal identification) known to the person and the investigator (CIOMS, p.17).

While confidentiality is an old concept in the treatment of a patient, it is a new and awkward concept in the surveillance of a population. The earliest surveillance programs – those of the 14th and 15th century Venetian Republic – were followed up with 40 days' quarantine, or exclusion from the Republic, both impossible outcomes if confidentiality was insisted upon. Later efforts at public health surveillance were either abstractive in nature (John Graunt's analysis of London Bills of Mortality in the 1660s; William Farr's death registration statistics in the 19th century) or stigmatizing (Rhode Island's 1741 law requiring tavern-keepers to report contagious disease among their patrons). However, it should be possible to comply with the patient-centered ethic of confidentiality without sacrificing the utility of tying blood test results to a particular person:

> At present, there is common recognition that the public interest may on certain occasion justify a breach of the principle of confidentiality, especially when the objective is to protect the health of the public (e.g., public health surveillance). For example, the medical profession in the countries of the European Economic Community generally accepts the following exceptions to the principle of confidentiality:
>
> - when there is a clear overriding duty to society;
> - when the information is required by law;
> - when the information is required for purposes of medical research and it is impractical or undesirable to seek explicit consent;
> - when the patient gives full, free and informed consent to disclosure.
>
> In Canada, the USA and many other countries, the public health laws provide similar exemptions to the principle of confidentiality—for such purposes as disease notification and certain public health interventions (Declich and Canter, p.289).

It should be clear that an important reason for GEOX to provide an actual health care station as part of its surveillance network, as opposed to just collecting blood samples "door-to-door," is to enjoy the best of both worlds in terms of confidentiality. The centralized blood testing laboratory can report coded results back to the health care practitioner who, in turn, can decode the name and notify the patient consistent with confidentiality. The GEOX surveillance network does not generally need to know the names of the patients on whom it has epidemiological data. And when it does need to know, a legitimate exception to confidentiality can probably be established. Via the coding system, GEOX can end up in contact with the patient, via their local health care practitioner.

Consequently, a global network of public health stations – where existing public health infrastructure is lacking – is not a utopian luxury in the context of xenotransplantation. It is a necessary element of a valid, normative regime. Similarly, the GEOX framework, while attractive, falls far short of a utopian dream. It lacks, for example, the characteristic "image of society's complete hold over those who belong to it" (*Utopia*, p.19). Individuals remain free not to participate in xenotransplantation at all, or not to visit basic health care stations established as part of the GEOX network. Even those infected with a xenogeneic virus, or thought to be susceptible to infection, will be brought under only as much social control (containment) as can be justified on the basis of avoiding direct threats to public health.

Interestingly, the very existence of xenotransplantation is somewhat contra-utopian because, as explained in chapter I, in a "perfect world" mandatory organ sharing among living people, and an "organ draft" upon death, would go a long way toward closing the organ gap. As utopia expert Rosabeth Kanter observes, "a communal vision assumes the best of people: that they are willing to sacrifice and share" (Kanter, p.237). Xenotransplantation needs to exist because people won't share their organs. GEOX needs to exist because, without it, xenotransplantation will be carried out selfishly (i.e., without due consideration of the risks to others) and ultimately to the detriment of the entire human population – by putting it at undue risk of xenozoonoses.

Financial Elements of a Global Xenotransplantation Control

The third geoethical principle set forth above, called the Assurance Principle, requires that new risks to global populations self-finance the means and methods of their risk management in accordance with globally-agreed norms. The moral force behind this principle is to avoid causing harm first with a modernization technology, and then inflicting economic losses as well when third parties are forced to bear the "clean-up costs" of the harm. In this section the costs and self-financeability of GEOX will be assessed. The aim is for GEOX to be a Maximal Competence organization similar to that arrived at via the preceding role-playing exercise. There are two basic cost elements associated with GEOX: certification processes (isolation), and global surveillance processes, including operation of health care stations in underdeveloped areas (containment).

Certification Costs are Minimal

A reasonable estimation of certification process costs can be achieved by estimating the number of xenotransplantation procedures that will be performed, the number of centers needed to perform those procedures, and a center-visitation frequency to ensure compliance with the promulgated norms. A fair starting point would seem to be one million xenograft procedures per year estimated in chapter I as the Euro-American latent demand. This represents more than a ten-fold increase over the number of procedures annually that can be accomplished with allografts, due to donor organ shortages.

It may further be reasonably assumed that each medical center performing such operations is able to accomplish, on average, three such procedures daily. This is the average rate that allotransplantation operates at today, without the convenience of having a transplantable xenograft "standing-by." Based on these two assumptions, GEOX would need to field adequate certification staff to monitor approximately one thousand xenograft programs.[2] Further assuming that each GEOX expert spends a week per program per year, there would be a need for 20 such experts.[3] Allotting 100% overhead for administrative and support personnel, and assuming an average, "fully loaded" cost of $200,000 per person per year, one arrives at a certification budget that is on the order of $8 million annually.[4] Within the administrative half of this budget there would be coverage of the donor herds and a continuing set of global meetings to iterate xenotransplantation norms.

Surveillance Costs are Basic Global Health Care Costs

A reasonable estimation of global surveillance processes can be achieved by estimating the cost of a health care station capable of providing primary care and performing blood tests, and multiplying that cost by the number of such stations needed to achieve an acceptable ratio of medic-per-persons worldwide. An actual doctor may not be needed on site to provide first-line health care (Basch, p.367), especially with use of satellite telemedicine technology (ASTP, p.ii). However, there are numerous other logical and efficient spin-off benefits to obtain from such health care stations, beyond serving as "friendly" blood-sampling outposts:

---

[2] (1,000,000 xenografts per year/(333 working days per year x 3 xenografts per day per program) = 1,000 programs).

[3] 1000 centers/50 weeklong visits per expert per year = 20 experts.

[4] (20 monitors + 20 administrative staff) x $200,000 per person fully-loaded cost = $8,000,000 annually.

- providing immunizations and preventative health information;
- offering maternal pre-natal care;
- assisting in the battle against antibiotic resistance, as described in chapter VII;
- performing with longitudinal cohort studies of different diseases over time

(Otten, pp.243; 247).

Consequently, another way to estimate the costs of the global surveillance prong of GEOX is to use figures developed by other expert organizations for the cost of performing the aforementioned spin-off benefits (Akin, p.17). Within the costs of providing these benefits, the additional expense of taking blood samples and sending them off for emerging disease analysis is likely to be quite small.

The World Bank has summarized its work in this area, and that of the WHO as follows (WDR is an abbreviation for World Development Report):

> In WDR93, the World Bank estimated that the cost of a basic package of clinical and public health services would be approximately US$12 per capita in low-income countries. In Better Health in Africa (1994), the Bank used a different methodology from the WDR to estimate the cost of such a package at around US$13 per capita in low-income and $16 per capita in middle-income African countries (Peters et al., p.16).

An earlier WHO estimate of $10 per capita to achieve "primary health care" in developing countries was developed as part of its Global Strategy for Health for All by the Year 2000, a program for the attainment "of a level of health that will permit [developing country persons] to lead a socially and economically productive life" (WHO 1999, p.viii.).

For the purposes of the surveillance prong of GEOX, the $10-$13 per capita figure should be applied to the number of people who lack access to primary health care facilities today. A good estimate of such a number is the number of people living in countries with per capita GNP below $1000 because nearly all unvaccinated children live in those countries (WHO 2000, p.83). That number of people totals, at most, 400 million (WHO 1999, pp.92-97).

In addition, it would be possible to estimate the number of people without primary health care according to those countries where the ratio of medical professionals to population falls below the minimal standard necessary to accomplish the primary health care mission (Beattie, p.142). A World Bank study has estimated that "in areas where poverty and malnutrition persist" successful accomplishment of primary health care requires bringing "worker/client ratios up to 1:1,000 or 1:1,500, even if this exceeds accepted national norms" (Heaver, p.21). Countries with major populations that have a ratio of doctors plus nurses to population below 1:1,500 include most of the African subcontinent, as well as Indonesia, the Philippines and Bangladesh (Beattie, p.142). Adding the populations of these countries, plus considering many countries of small population in deep poverty, a reasonable estimate population of a multiplier as for the per capita primary health care factor is 1 billion people. To obtain a high-end estimate, we will use the highest per capita figure developed by the World Bank, $13 per person for a basic package of clinical and public health services in a low-income developing country.

Consequently, $13 billion per year is the approximate cost of the surveillance (containment) prong of GEOX's health care mission. It is justified as including the costs of providing annual primary health care to people living in countries with either less than $1000 per capita GNP or less than a 1:1,500 ratio of doctors plus nurses to population. Clearly, it is this prong of the GEOX mission that dominates its cost. Compared to the disease surveillance costs, the costs of xenograft certification are immaterial. If instead global health care needs to include many more people, and the cost is much more than $13 billion, then the higher cost must be supported in order for xenotransplantation to proceed.

The $13 billion budget derived above would fund about 650,000 health care stations at a ratio of one station per 1,500 inhabitants for the billion most health care deprived people in the world. This works out to an average budget of about $20,000 per health care station per year. That budget would have to cover the costs of a health care staff (training and salaries), basic medicines and vaccines, and infrastructure support (building, power, communications, supplies). However, several studies have shown that modest fee-for-service arrangements do not detract from public use of health care facilities, even in the poorest countries (World Bank, pp.25-48). Consequently, the aforementioned budget could even be supplemented with fee-for-service arrangements for non-basic care.

The GEOX budget would also enable bulk drug purchases that could substantially reduce pharmaceutical costs in developing countries. The organization Medicins Sans Frontieres has created emergency drug kits that are designed to provide the key pharmaceutical needs of 10,000 people for three months (Pinel, p.218). The organization has also paved the way in showing that bulk drug purchases can reduce per unit costs substantially, although drug company cooperation is obviously needed as well (Pecoul et al., p.363).

The Xenograft Tax

With GEOX expenditures of approximately $13 billion annually, and the geoethical Assurance Principle requirement that xenotransplantation itself bear the burden of this cost, there would be a necessary "xenograft tax" to GEOX of $13,000 per organ at the demand rate shown in chapter I to be one million operations per year.[5] Such a cost is, in fact, quite modest compared to the cost of allotransplantation procedures in the United States today – about 5 percent of the

---

[5] ($13 billion dollars/1,000,000 procedures per year = $13,000 per procedure).

cost of a heart transplant. While this cost is about 50 percent of the average United Kingdom transplantation fee, it must be recalled that such a fee includes the cost of procuring the organ from a cadaveric patient, generally at the scene of a highway accident. These "organ harvesting" fees would be unnecessary when xenografts were used, although there would remain the need to compensate the xenograft-growing company and the medical care team at the hospital.

The xenograft tax would be most logically levied on the pharmaceutical companies selling the xenografts, as a kind of global sales tax. While any sales tax on pharmaceuticals has the effect of reducing demand, the amount of that reduction is directly proportional to the elasticity of demand (Jacobs, p.288). If demand is very sensitive to price, then the effect of a sales tax could be to "kill the golden goose" because nearly all demand would dry up. On the other hand, if the demand curve is vertical, or nearly so, then a sales tax has almost no effect on demand.

There is little evidence that organ transplantation has an elastic demand curve within a broad range of prices. After all, the price of a transplant is ten times higher in the United States than the United Kingdom, and yet the market will pay for all the transplants that can be done. Instead, because transplants are almost always monopoly products due to legal controls, and because there are, by definition, no substitute products when an organ transplant is needed, demand is highly inelastic in the vertical direction. Consequently, negotiations with government agencies or a few major third-party insurance payors tend to set prices at the unnecessarily often quite high value of chronic hospitalization, the next best alternative. Therefore, it is unlikely that a xenograft sales tax imposed on pharmaceutical companies will diminish the projected demand of one million xenografts per year.

In any event, at least in accordance with this role-playing exercise, the $13,000 per xenograft GEOX tax is a fair approximation of the price of managing the global risks imposed by xenotransplantation. To recast the solution in both economic *and* global risk terms, a $13,000 per xenograft GEOX tax is the price of obtaining the "approval of all affected in their capacity as participants in a practical discourse," which, in turn, is the threshold condition that must be met before "norms can claim to be valid" (Habermas, p.66). This remains the case even in the event that surveillance and global health care costs are much higher than $13 billion, and a GEOX tax of more than $13,000 is called for.

As to the First World health care payors who complain about why *they* should shoulder the costs of health care in the Third World, there is no truer response than "enlightened self interest." In a recent editorial entitled *Preventing Disease: We're All In This Together*, the Chairman of the U.S. House of Representatives International Relations Committee, Benjamin Gilman, pleaded for G-7 involvement in the health care systems of developing countries. He cited the mounting liability the United States faces due to "the heavy cost that international infectious diseases impose" (Gilman and Gejdenson, p.6). He also noted that the U.S. spends more than $230 million annually on polio vaccinations domestically, solely because polio has not been eliminated from the developing world.

Infectious diseases that fester overseas will be on First World doorsteps at the speed and volume of international air travel.

Finally, from a financial standpoint, it might be argued that if the First World can afford billions of dollars for xenografts, and billions of dollars for xenograft taxes, why not simply allocate billions of dollars for Third World health care and avoid creating the new xenogeneic disease risks associated with xenotransplantation? Why not directly allocate foreign aid funds for Third World health care rather than providing such financing via a tax on xenografts? The principal answer to these questions is that few things get accomplished in political arenas that are not forced. Lobbies for health care in developing countries have never commanded the power of lobbies for military assistance to strategic countries. The West can, of course, *afford* to establish a global basic health care capability in the developing world. It has just never been a *priority*, probably because (1) the people in developing countries who lack health care are among the most disempowered constituencies in the world, (2) global health care advocates in the West have failed to organize sufficient political power to direct budgetary spending, and (3) diseases emerging from developing countries have not yet become infective enough in the West to challenge social stability, and hence impact budget priorities.

However, there is a subsidiary answer to why a xenograft tax is a more sensible means of accomplishing basic global health care than national budgetary grants. To understand this answer it is important to first clearly lay out the flow of funds from a xenograft tax:

- a tax of $13,000 per xenograft sold is levied on the selling pharmaceutical company, and is payable directly to GEOX;
- GEOX uses the tax funds to pay the expenses of its xenograft certification teams, to pay the expenses of in-country basic health care stations (established in a rational sequence based on need and feasibility) and to pay the expenses of managing a global registry of xenograft recipients and a global waiting list for developing country access to 5-10 percent of xenotransplantation procedures;
- pharmaceutical companies charge health care payors (e.g. governments or health insurance companies) a fee for each xenograft, which includes the tax it paid on it;
- health care payors indirectly pass on the costs to the general public via general taxes or health insurance premiums;
- effectively, individuals in xenotransplanting countries pay a slightly larger percentage of their disposable income for health care services by virtue of the availability of xenotransplantation and the concomitant obligation of funding basic health care worldwide via a xenograft tax.

Now, the benefit of this process is that responsibility for establishing and operating the basic health care stations rests firmly with GEOX, an international organization with a clear mission. This addresses one of the biggest bugaboos blocking Western funding for Third World health care services today – fear that the monies will be wasted. The waste can arise as much from the bureaucratic restrictions of government-to-government funding as it can from misallocations within the recipient country. In either event, these sources of waste are eliminated with GEOX-operated facilities.

The political "forcing function" for this solution will arise when Western countries ask developing countries to forego national xenotransplantation procedures that don't meet Western standards, and to permit intrusive bio-surveillance of their populations for emerging disease threats. Developing countries will likely respond that, to do so, they must be promised access to Western xenotransplantation procedures, and they must be provided with a practical and ethical means of carrying out bio-surveillance (Leary, "Defining," p.46). GEOX funded with a xenograft tax is, therefore, a uniquely viable financial solution to developed and developing country interests in the xenobiology arena. Its global basic health care mission permits bio-surveillance to be conducted both practically and ethically, i.e., epidemiology accompanied by treatment (CIOMS, p.15). And yet its financing does not worsen the budget crisis of any country. Indeed, were GEOX to be (1) chartered as a private international organization, (2) given the exclusive right to collect the xenograft tax in exchange for performing the GEOX duties, as described above, and (3) permitted to retain any surplus as a dividend pool for its shareholders, then such an organization may be able to raise substantial investment funds upfront, in advance of the implementation of xenotransplantation, and thereby get a "head-start" on its GEOX tasks.

Legal Pathways to a Global Xenotransplantation Control

The practical implementation of GEOX requires that a treaty be signed and ratified by as many countries as possible, and certainly all countries capable of supporting xenotransplantation services. Treaties are the documents that evidence a legally-binding and internationally-enforceable obligation upon countries to do or not do certain things. In the case of GEOX, countries are needed to ensure that organizations and individuals within their jurisdiction comply with the Maximum Competence norms governing xenotransplantation. Consequently, the key question here is how can a GEOX Treaty most plausibly come into force?

A GEOX Treaty can achieve its validity only by being authored, with full discourse participation, by the same entities to which it will apply and affect. These "Janus faces that law turns toward its addressees on the one side and its authors on the other" (Habermas, *Between*, p.129) are the *sine qua non* of valid norms, and also prescribe the legal pathway for norm development. Consequently it is necessary for a GEOX Treaty to flow from one or more "norm-setting" meetings of all affected parties. The convocation of such meetings will also accomplish the important task of providing global notice that there is an agenda for change:

> The task of change is to arouse expectations on the part of as many effective participants as possible that they will be relatively better off in terms of net value position by paying the costs necessary to substitute genuine inclusive public order for disorder among parochial orders (McDougal et al., p.1091).

Some one or more entities needs to commence the treaty-making process with an alert to the world that it is at risk of "disorder among parochial orders," due to the advent of xenotransplantation. This alert would emphasize that it is in the world's interest to ensure "effective participation" at a series of treaty-preparatory meetings empowered to create a "genuine inclusive public order" for the new medical technology. The alert could then set a schedule for treaty-preparatory meetings, and provide a means for registration. An effective alert would be published in multiple journals, and be sponsored by respected organizing entities.

Sentinel Organizations

The sentinel organizing entities could come from professional organizations such as the International Xenotransplantation Association or International Society of Heart and Lung Transplantation,[6] since they are highly aware of the issue. Alternatively, the organizing entity could be an intergovernmental organization such as the World Health Organization, a business organization involved in transplantation such as Novartis, or a non-profit health organization such as the Red Cross. Individual countries could take the lead such as one with a technological headstart in xenotransplantation (e.g., the Interim Xenotransplantation Authority or the Centers for Disease Control), one with much to gain due to low allotransplantation rates (e.g., Russian or Japanese Foreign Ministries). Finally, it could even be issue-oriented non-governmental organizations (NGOs) that take the lead, such as the Canadian Heart Association or a major religion. The benefit of a new GEOX is that it starts with a "clean slate." This, in itself, will be of great benefit for the complicated undertaking of establishing a global public health surveillance and xenotransplantation certification system.

---

[6] In December 2000, the ISHLT issued preemptory recommendations that call for a moratorium on animal-to-human organ transplants until (a) microbiologists agree that the xenogeneic risks are minimal, (b) primate studies have provided convincing evidence of safety and efficacy, (c) national regulatory structures are empowered, and (d) an international registry of xenograft recipients is in place (Cooper 2000 et al., p.1144).

Participation Sectors

A decision-making process fully consistent with global consensus ethics is necessary to achieve progress toward a treaty. The best solution to this dilemma lies in representative democracy: representatives of different key "participation sectors" achieve consensus among themselves, while the representatives are informed by super-majority voting within their own "participation sector." Logical participation sectors for xenotransplantation could include:

Table VII-1 Geoethical Participation Sectors

Power-Granting Participation Sectors

1) High-Income Countries (e.g., U.K., U.S.)

2) Medium-Income Countries (e.g., China, India)

3) Low-Income Countries (e.g., Ethiopia, Cambodia)

Knowledge-Granting Participation Sectors

4) Professional Associations (e.g., Medical Unions, Law Societies)

5) Business Organizations (e.g., Pharmaceutical Companies)

6) Non-Profit Health Organizations (e.g., Medicins San Frontiers)

Compliance-Granting Participation Sectors

7) Intergovernmental Organizations (e.g., WHO, WTO, UNESCO)

8) Religious Organizations (e.g., Church of England, Vatican)

9) Other NGOs (e.g., People for Ethical Treatment of Animals)

The treaty-making process would proceed initially via 3-9 separate preparatory meetings within each participation sector, or a set of three authority-related participation sectors. At such meetings there would be education, Habermasian discourse, adopted platforms, and an elected representative to the ultimate treaty-writing meeting. Subsequently, a larger simultaneous meeting of all participation sectors could occur, and within this larger meeting, representatives of each participation sector could meet and, via practical Habermasian discourse, arrive at a consensus treaty text. The benefit of having the nine representatives meet within the larger context of all participation sector participants is to provide a continuous flow of input to the representatives from the participation sector constituencies that they represent.

Once a treaty text is adopted, it will be necessary for the Power-Granting Participation Sector entities to utilize their national processes to achieve ratification of the treaty. This difficult process will be facilitated by virtue of the active participation of sovereign governments in the treaty-development process (via their participation sector), as well as the participation of other non-governmental organizations such as professional associations, private companies, public health groups and religious orders. Upon ratification of the treaty by a requisite number of States, GEOX will come into force. Its authority and effectiveness will grow as more national ratifications are received, as xenotransplantation programs become certified, and as GEOX tax revenues commence funding global health surveillance stations.

Enforcement of GEOX rules will be provided for in the treaty text. The enforcement provisions can be expected to have logical nexuses to the disease isolation and containment mission. These sanctions would proceed in an escalating manner, such as (1) public warnings, (2) suspension of access to certified xenotransplantation programs for rogue country, (3) restrictions on air travel with the rogue country, and (4) quarantine until medical clearance of persons believed to have visited the rogue country.

The entire legal pathway to GEOX can be plausibly mapped out as follows:

Year 1 – Sentinel participants organize themselves:

- at their own annual meetings and/or via correspondence.

Year 2 – Sentinel participants converge on the basics:

- "strawman" treaty to serve as a focus for discussions;
- a meeting schedule for participation sectors;
- obtaining "seed funding" to cover start-up expenses.

Year 3 – Sentinel participants announce a schedule of meetings:

- "strawman" treaty provisions and information distributed;
- announcement is made in many major publications.

Year 4 – Intra-sector participant meetings held per registration procedures:

- positions adopted on "strawman" treaty provisions;
- sector representative elected by super-majority voting.

Year 5 – All sector participant meeting to finalize GEOX treaty:

- decisions taken by practical discourse among nine representatives;
- decisions informed by continuous input from all participants.

Year 6 – National treaty ratifications occur and GEOX is formed.

Year 7 – Consolidation of GEOX.

Year 8 – Certifications and global health care stations commence.

Of course the schedule and substance set forth above are purely exemplary in nature. They are meant to show that the theoretical solutions to the conflict between private and public interests in xenotransplantation explored in this book are, in fact, solvable in a practical manner. Consequently, under this schedule, no xenotransplantation outside of strictly controlled experimental protocols with very few patients should occur for the next eight years.

Not the First Time the Rich Tax Themselves for Global Benefit

The potential practicality of GEOX can be seen by the fact that it would not be the first world organization empowered to control an important aspect of human affairs. That path was pioneered with the formation of the International Telegraph Union (now the International Telecommunication Union) in 1866, an organization empowered to control global use of electromagnetic frequencies. It was widened substantially in the aftermath of World War II via numerous UN-affiliated bodies, and embellished in the 1980s and 1990s with entities such as the mineral wealth distributing International Seabed Authority and the import/export competent World Trade Organization. GEOX simply extends this century of precedent to the realm of hybrid human-animal biosystems.

A particularly appropriate precedent for GEOX is the Intelsat Organization, formed between 1965 and 1971 for the purpose of enabling a global satellite communications service. It was appreciated at the time that satellite communications would only be maximally beneficial if most countries participated in the satellite network. However, most countries could not afford to help pay for launching satellites, or even to install satellite ground stations (which had to be certified as meeting demanding technical specifications) in their major cities. Furthermore, since the day-to-day functions of satellite communications are operational in nature – not political – it was thought that a non-governmental organization rather than an inter-governmental organization should take responsibility.

To solve the dilemma of a few rich countries needing global buy-in, a treaty was signed between countries to create a non-government organization in which the wealthier countries paid almost all of the costs, and were entitled to use almost all of the capacity of the satellite system (Intelsat, article V). These funds provided the means for poorer countries to install national ground stations. Thus wealthier countries gained the significant benefit (especially to multinational corporations) of being able to send satellite messages anywhere in the world, while poorer countries gained the benefit of having some access to a global communications network. In essence, the wealthier countries were taxed on their use of globally-regulated outer space orbits and electromagnetic spectrum frequencies in order to enable some use of those orbits and frequencies by poorer countries.

The Intelsat experience is directly analogous to the proposal herein of taxing wealthier countries on their use of the life-extending capability of xenotransplantation in order to enable some life-extending capability in the poorer countries, both via queued access to xenotransplantation procedures and direct access to basic health care services. The wealthier countries will gain the significant benefit (especially to multinationals) of having a healthier, and safer, world to dwell within. The poorer countries will gain the major benefit of relatively large increases in life expectancy associated with basic health care services. Furthermore, it is a new international organization that will be meeting the needs of both the poor and rich countries, which bypasses the suspicions and politics that loom larger with direct State action. Indeed, the signatories to the Intelsat Agreement also promised to avoid participating in rogue satellite systems that would cause significant economic harm to the new International Organization (Intelsat, Art. XIV). An analogous undertaking will be needed for GEOX, albeit with respect to precluding rogue xenotransplantation operations (Kumar, p.628). The following table identifies a path for GEOX that parallels the successful Intelsat experience:

Table VII-2 Comparison of International Telecommunications Satellite Organization and Proposed Global Enforcement Organization for Xenobiology

	INTELSAT	**GEOX**
Charter:	A Treaty	A Treaty
Owners:	National PT&T's	National Health Depts
Restriction:	1 Owner/Country	1 Owner/Country
Exclusivity:	Every Country	Every Country
Investment:	Proportional to Satellite Use	Proportional to Xenograft Use
If Too Poor:	Granted a Token Ownership	Granted a Token Ownership
Benefits:	Global Satellite Access	Access to Xenografts
Obligation:	Permit Intelsat Earth Station;	Permit GEOX Health Stations;
	Comply With Specifications;	Comply With Regulations;
	Don't Hurt Intelsat Business	Don't Disturb GEOX Regime
Dividends:	Paid Based on Investment	Paid Based on Investment
Voting:	Policies: 1 Country, 1 Vote	Policies: 1 Country, 1 Vote
	Operations: Per Investment	Operations: Per Investment

Although it has been necessary for Intelsat to invest billions of dollars in launching satellites, after several years the organization began paying regular dividends to its members, which are largely government telecommunications departments. A management-like "secretariat" runs the organization on a day-to-day basis, and reports periodically to both an Assembly (with one seat per country) and to a Board of Governors (elected on the basis of the owners' share of the investment capital).

It is important to note that, initially, the Intelsat Treaty had only a dozen signatories, but, by its terms, was always open for new countries to join. Over the following two decades, nearly every country in the world did sign the treaty and become a member of the Intelsat Organization. Similarly, GEOX can begin with just a few countries; the inherent attractiveness of having access to xenotransplantation procedures may be a sufficient "carrot" to induce global membership. On the other hand, there are many differences between 21st century xenotransplantation and mid-20th century satellite communications. GEOX would certainly be more effective if it aimed for near-global membership from the very beginning.

Conclusion

It has been shown in this chapter that the substantive financial and legal elements of a global enforcement organization for xenobiology are practically achievable. Indeed, many of the elements have direct precedents in regimes established for outer space, the electromagnetic spectrum, and the international seabed. What is most important to remember, however, is that xenotransplantation only makes geoethical sense via a concomitantly established global enforcement regime. If this regime is absent, then xenotransplantation should not proceed. Barry Commoner is right in claiming that, in biology, as in economics, there is no such thing as a "free lunch" (Commoner, *The Closing*, p.46). The costs of xenotransplantation are high, but the value of life is much higher still. If society is unwilling to incur the costs of GEOX, then it cannot morally breach the barrier of xenobiology.

Chapter VIII

Summary

This book commenced with a factual demonstration of an outstanding need for additional vital organs to use in transplantation procedures. It was shown that the demand for vital organs is significantly understated in published reports. The understatement arises from *a priori* screening criteria that aim to keep waiting lists in rough consistency with the supply of allografts from cadaveric and living donors. In fact, a latent demand for millions of organs exists, a demand far beyond the capability of voluntary organ donation systems to satisfy, especially for the human heart.

While a variety of technologies are in development to address both the extant and latent demand for transplantable organs, xenotransplantation technology appears to be the technology closest to fruition. It also has the benefit, as compared to biomechanical solutions, of being more "forgettable" by the patients. Even if the near future boasts a competitive mix of organ replacement technologies, it is probable that a large share of the market will be garnered by xenografts.

The future of xenotransplantation has been shadowed with ethical concerns. Animal care advocates are troubled by the destruction of animal lives for human medical benefit, and public health advocates worry about the creation of new human diseases via the inadvertent xenotransplantation of animal viruses. On the other hand there is a solid case to be made that sick people have a *right* to a xenograft if it could save their life. This right is not absolute, with its principle conditions being national affordability and public health safety.

This book showed that the conflict between private and public interests in xenotransplantation is capable of resolution. Animal care interests are addressable via xenograft breeding practices that are sensitive to that which we believe pigs appreciate. This means avoidance of pain and stressful living conditions for the pigs. National budget limitations may limit the availability of xenotransplantation, but should not ethically proscribe the treatment for at least some who can benefit from it. Public health concerns are addressable via applicability to xenotransplantation of the type of isolation and containment procedures that were agreed upon at the Asilomar Conference for the management of genetically modified organisms.

The application of Asilomar-type procedures to xenotransplantation requires an extended analysis because of the probability that any harmful xenozoonotic viruses would escape from one country into the global public health environment. This means that a quasi-communitarian ethical process will be needed to achieve "buy-in" to xenotransplantation from all those who are at risk from its dangers.

The likely outcome of globally participative norm-setting will be a new Global Enforcement Organization for Xenotransplantation, abbreviated GEOX. The role of GEOX in xenotransplantation would include certification that xenograft herds and transplant centers complied with Asilomar-type risk isolation and containment rules. In order to carry out this role, in a global environment that includes many countries without effective health care systems, GEOX must assume responsibility for emerging disease surveillance in such countries. Such a responsibility can only be accomplished by tasking GEOX with the frank provision of a basic health care capability in those countries.

The book has estimated the rough order of magnitude of the cost of implementing health care stations throughout underserved developing countries at approximately $13 billion annually. While this is a large number in general, it is only about 1 percent of health care spending in the United States. Furthermore, it can be self-financed via a $13,000 tax on each xenograft transplanted, assuming one million xenotransplantations are conducted annually. The $13,000 tax is well within the transplantation spending envelope currently assumed for allografts. Even with the much greater spending on transplantation that would occur with xenotransplantation, due to much greater organ availability, total health care spending in developed countries would remain within a few percent of their current levels.

Modernization technologies such as xenotransplantation tend to create global risks that, in turn, propel national societies into global arrangements in order to effectuate risk management schemes. The norms that result from global risk management derive their validity from a communitarian process of practical discourse among all affected participants. In fact, the very process of global risk management involves the synthesis of communitarian values from a world community brought together by new risks exploding in their midst. Geoethics is a new philosophical outlook to guide the new communitarian synthesis. Geoethics is an extrapolation to world affairs of applied philosophies conceived in terms of subjects as individuals. The core principles of geoethics are:

- Conduct only those activities of potential global effect that promote the greatest relative fulfillment of basic human needs in the most distressed parts of the world (Benefit Principle);
- Implement activities of potential global effect only in such manner as achieves the consent of all parties who may be adversely affected by such activities, through their representatives (Risk Principle);
- Activities of potential global effect must self-finance the means and methods of independent assurance of their compliance with global norms (Assurance Principle).

The GEOX regime proposed in this book resolves the conflict between private and public interests in xenotransplantation consistently with the principles of geoethics. As to the Benefit Principle, the greatest beneficiaries of the new norms will be those persons in the least developed countries who will achieve some satisfaction of their basic need for health care, paid for by a tax on xenografts. The Risk Principle is achieved because the norms will be adopted and modified via a regime that includes participation of all affected parties – governmental, nongovernmental and intergovernmental organizations, professional, business and public health associations, and wealthy, modest and poor constituencies. Finally, the risky consequences of xenotransplantation globally are managed with self-generated funds, through the GEOX tax, in compliance with the Assurance Principle.

Resolution of the conflict between private and public interests in xenotransplantation requires a large undertaking. However, the benefit of such a project is to take human health care to a new level of optimization, both in wealthy countries and in those that have a severe shortage of resources. The geoethical task is therefore justified by its promotion of the basic human need for health. Satisfaction of this need, it will be recalled, is the most fundamental prerequisite for participation in the very society that constitutes, in its endless quest for improvement, the *raison d'etre* Kant envisioned as "the destined final end, the highest moral perfection to which the human race can attain" (Kant, p.253).

Xenotransplantation, implemented via geoethical principles, promises to make the world a much better place. But xenotransplantation without geoethics is a reckless thing to do. Ultimately, it is at just such a locus that the objectives of philosophy, medicine and social science intersect. When the ethics are missing, the procedure must stop. No ends ever justify any means necessary. *Consequently, xenotransplantation should not proceed in advance of a global enforcement regime for xenobiology*. This is not a stultification of progress. It is, on the contrary, an impetus for success.

Within a handful of years it would be practically possible to create a global enforcement organization for xenobiology. Such an organization will ensure global buy-in to risk minimization standards and a just allocation of global resources spent on xenobiology. Certainly a brief pause for greater safety, and global harmony, is wiser than a rush toward possible danger, and worldwide dissension. This wisdom resolves the conflict between private and public interests in xenotransplantation, and opens the door to a major expansion of longevity and quality of life.

Bibliography

Abouna, G. "The Use of Ex Vivo Xenogeneic Whole Liver Perfusion as a Bridge to Liver Regeneration or Liver Transplantation." *Graft* 4 (2001): 120-25.

Ahuja, A. "Progress, or crimes against nature?" *The Times*, 8 Oct. 1999, sec. 3: 36.

Akin, J. *Financing Health Services in Developing Countries: An Agenda for Reform.* Washington, D.C.: World Bank, 1999 ed.

Allan, J. *Financing Health Services in Developing Countries: An Agenda for Reform.* Washington, D.C.: World Bank, 1999 ed.

American Medical Association. *Family Medical Guide*. New York: Random House, 1982.

Animal-to-Human Transplants: The Ethics of Xenotransplantation. London: Nuffield Council on Bioethics, 1996.

Appell, D. "The New Uncertainty Principle." *Scientific American*, Jan. 2001: 18-19.

Appleyard, Bryan. "The Mad Forces of Genetic Darkness." *The Sunday Times, London*, 21 Feb. 1999: 17.

Ascher, N. "Cadaver Organ Shortages: Present Alternatives." *Organ Procurement, Preservation and Distribution in Transplantation*. Ed. M. Phillips. Richmond, VA: UNOS, 1996.

ASTP, *1999 Report on U.S. Telemedicine Activity*. Ed. Grigsby, B., 2000.

"Avian Viruses Reemerge as Threat." *Scientific American Medicine Bulletin*. Ed. D. Federman. 22 (1999): 5.

"Baboon Liver Passes Virus to Man." 30 September 1999. http://www.cnn.com.

Bach, F. "Putting the Public at Risk." *Bulletin of the World Health Organization* 77.1 (1999): 65-68.

Barinaga, M. "Asilomar Revisited: Lessons for Today?" *Science* 287 (2000): 1584.

Basch, P. *Textbook of International Health.* 2nd ed. New York: Oxford University Press, 1999.

Beattie, ed. *Sustainable Health Care Financing in Southern Africa: Papers from an EDI Health Policy Seminar held in Johannesburg, South Africa*. Washington, D.C.: World Bank, 1998.

Beauchamp, T. and James F. Childress. *Principles of Biomedical Ethics*. 4th ed. New York: Oxford University Press, 1994.

Beck, U. *Risk Society: Towards a New Modernity*, London: Sage, 1992.

Becker, Y. "Use of Marginal Donors in Kidney Transplantation." *Graft* (2000)3: 216-20.

Bentham, J. *An Introduction to the Principles of Morals And Legislation*. 1789. Oxford: Basil Blackwell, 1960.

Berlin, I. *Four Essays on Liberty*. Oxford: Oxford University Press, 1969.

--- *The Power of Ideas*. Ed. H. Hardy. Princeton: Princeton University Press, 2000.

Bioartificial Organs: Science, Medicine and Technology. Ed. A. Prokop et al. New York: New York Academy of Sciences, 1997. 127-37.

Bloom, B. "The Future of Public Health." *Nature*. 402 (Dec. 1999): C63.

Bloor, D. *Wittgenstein: A Social Theory of Knowledge*. New York: McMillan, 1983.

Blumberg, B. *Hepatitis B: The Hunt for a Killer Virus*. Princeton, NJ: Princeton University Press, 2002.

--- "Bioethical Questions Related to Hepatitis B Antigen." *American Journal of Clinical Pathology* 65 (1976): 848-53.

Blumberg, B. and R. Fox. "The Daedalus Effect: Changes in Ethical Questions Relating to Hepatitis B Virus." *Annals of Internal Medicine*. 102 (1985): 390-394.

Bollinger, R. and O. Salvatierra. "The Future of Transplantation." *Organ Procurement, Preservation and Distribution in Transplantation*. Ed. M. Phillips. Richmond, VA: UNOS, 1996. 411-18.

Brazelton, T. and A. Cheung. "Pharmacologic Immunosuppressants in Xenotransplantation." *Xenotransplantation: The Transplantation of Organs and Tissues Between Species*. Ed. D.K.C. Cooper. 2nd ed. Berlin: Springer, 1997. 736-48.

"Brazil Launches New Initiative to Increase Organ Donation." *Transplant News*, 16 March 2001.

"Briefing: Xenotransplantation." *Nature* 391 (1998): 6665.

Brody, E. *Biomedical Technology and Human Rights*. Cambridge: University Press, 1993.

Bronsther, O. "The Dialectic Nature of Xenotransplantation." *Journal of the American College of Surgeons* 186.4 (1998): 397-401.

Brown, D. "New Study Links Deadly 1918 Flu to Virus in Birds." *The Washington Post*, 23 May 2000: A19.

Buhler, L. et al. "Xenotransplantation – State of the Art – Update 1999." *Frontiers in Bioscience* 4 (1999): 416-32.

Butler, J. *The Ethics of Health Care Rationing: Principles and Practices*. London: Cassell Publishing, 1999.

Callender, C. "Educational Aspects of Organ Procurement." *Organ Procurement, Preservation and Distribution in Transplantation*. Ed. M. Phillips. Richmond, VA: UNOS, 1996. 347-56.

Calva, J., et al. "Antibiotic Usage and Antibiotic Resistance in Latin America." *Antibiotic Resistance: From Molecular Basics to Therapeutic Options*. Ed. Amabile-Cuevas. Austin: R.G. Landes Company, 1996. 73-97.

Cannon, G. *Superbug: Nature's Revenge*. London: Virgin Publishing, 1995.

Caplan, A. "The case for using pigs," *Bulletin of the World Health Organization*. 77.1 (1999): 67-69.

--- *If I Were A Rich Man Could I Buy A Pancreas?* Bloomington, IN: Indiana University Press, 1992.

Cassileth, B. et al. "Understanding Public Attitudes to Clinical Xenotransplantation." *Graft* 4 (2001):146-48.

Cate, F. "Human Organ Transplantation: The Role of Law." *The Journal of Corporation Law*, Fall 1994: 69-90.

Cavalli-Sforza, L. et al. *The History and Geography of Human Genes*. Princeton: Princeton University Press, 1994.

Chang, R. "Artificial Cells and Bioencapsulation in Bioartificial Organs." *Bioartificial Organs: Science, Medicine and Technology*. Ed. A. Prokop et al. New York: New York Academy of Sciences, 1997. 249-59.

Chapman, L. and J. Fishman. "Xenotransplantation and Infectious Diseases." *Xenotransplantation: The Transplantation of Organs and Tissues Between Species*. Ed. D.K.C. Cooper et. al. 2nd ed. Berlin: Springer, 1997. 736-48.

Chapman, L. "Speculation, Stringent Reasoning and Science." *Bulletin of the World Health Organization* 77.1 (1999): 68-70.

Chen, S. et al. "Treatment of Severe Liver Failure with a Bioartificial Liver." *Bioartificial Organs: Science, Medicine and Technology*. Ed. A. Prokop et al. New York: New York Academy of Sciences, 1997. 350-60.

Childress, J.F. "Ethical Criteria for Procuring and Distributing Organs for Transplantation." *Organ Transplantation Policy: Issues and Prospects*. Eds. J. Blumenstein and F. Sloan. Durham: Duke University Press, 1989. 87-113.

CIOMS. *International Guidelines for Ethical Review of Epidemiological Studies*. Geneva: WHO, 1991.

Clark, M. "This Little Piggy Went to Market: The Xenotransplantation and Xenozoonoses Debate." *The Journal of Law, Medicine & Ethics* 27 (1999): 137-52.

"Clinical Islet Xenotransplantation – Transplantation of Porcine Islets into Diabetic Patients." *Xenotransplantation: The Transplantation of Organs and Tissues Between Species*. Ed. D.K.C. Cooper. 2nd ed. Berlin: Springer, 1997. 812-20.

Cohen, M. "Changing Patterns of Infectious Disease." *Nature* 406 (2000): 762-67.

--- "Epidemiological Factors Influencing the Emergence of Antimicrobial Resistance." *Antibiotic Resistance: Origins, Evolution, Selection and Spread*. New York: John Wiley & Sons, 1997. 223-37.

Coleman, P. "Brother, Can You Spare a Liver? Five Ways to Increase Organ Donation." *Valparaiso University Law Review* 31 (1996): 1-41.

Commoner, B. *Science & Survival*. 1963. New York: Viking Press, 1967.

--- *The Closing Circle: Nature, Man and Technology*. New York: Knopf, 1971.

Cooper, D. and R. Lanza. *Xeno: The Promise of Transplanting Animal Organs into Humans*. Oxford: Oxford University Press, 2000.

Cooper, D. et al. "Report of the Xenotransplantation Advisory Committee of the International Society for Heart and Lung Transplantation: The Present Status of Xenotransplantation and its Potential Role in the Treatment of End-Stage Cardiac and Pulmonary Diseases." *Journal of Heart and Lung Transplantation* 19 (2000): 1125-61.

Council on Ethical and Judicial Affairs, American Medical Association. "Financial Incentives for Organ Procurement: Ethical Aspects of Future Contracts for Cadaveric Donors." *Archives of Internal Medicine* 155 (1995): 581-89.

Cozzi, E. et al. "Effect of Transgentic Expression of Human Decay-Accelerating Factor on the Inhibition of Hyperacute Rejection of Pig Organs." *Xenotransplantation: The Transplantation of Organs and Tissues Between Species*. Ed. D.K.C. Cooper. 2nd ed. Berlin: Springer, 1997. 677.

Culpepper, M. "Legal Aspects of Organ and Tissue Procurement and Transplantation." *Organ Procurement, Preservation and Distribution in Transplantation*. Ed. M. Phillips. Richmond, VA: UNOS, 1996. 347-56.

Daar, A.S. "Animal-to-Human Transplants – A Solution or a New Problem?" *Bulletin of the World Health Organization* 77.1 (1999): 54-61.

--- "Choosing Risk-Benefit Analysis or Precautionary Principle as Our Approach to Clinical Xenotransplantation." *Graft* 4 (2001): 164-66.

Data Highlights from the 1998 Annual Report of the U.S. Scientific Registry of Transplant Recipients and the Organ Procurement and Transplantation Network. Washington, D.C.: Department of Health and Human Services, 1998.

Davis, J., ed. *Managed Care Systems and Emerging Infections: Challenges and Opportunities for Strengthening Surveillance, Research, and Prevention*, Washington D.C.: Institute of Medicine Forum on Emerging Infections, National Academy Press, 2000.

De Waal, F. and F. Lanting. *Bonobo: The Forgotten Ape*, Berkeley: University of California Press, 1997.

"Deaths and Death Rates for the 10 Leading Causes of Death in Specified Age Groups: United States." *National Vital Statistics Report*. Vol. 47, No. 4, Table 17. Washington, D.C.: Department of Health and Human Services, 1998.

Decision Adopted by the Conference of the Parties to the Convention on Biological Diversity at the Resumed Session of its First Extraordinary Meeting, 24-29 January 2000, Montreal. Cartagena Biosafety Protocol, 2000.

Declich, S. and A.O. Carter. "Public Health Surveillance: Historical Origins, Methods and Evaluation." *Bulletin of the World Health Organization*, 72.2 (1994): 285-304.

"Despite Legislative Ban, Selling Organs for Transplantation Continues to Thrive in India." *Transplant News*, 16 March 2001.

"Diacrin, Beth Israel Deaconess Report Conducting First Fetal Pig Cell Transplant in Brain of Stroke Patient." *Transplant News*, 31 October 1999.

Ditlea, S. "Change of Heart." *Red Herring*. Oct. 2002, 28.

Doyal, L. "Medical Ethics and Moral Indeterminacy." *Journal of Law and Society*. 17 (1990): 1-16.

--- "Needs, Rights, and Equity: Moral Quality in Healthcare Rationing." *Quality in Health Care* 4 (1995): 273-83.

--- "Public Participation and the Moral Quality of Healthcare Rationing." *Quality in Health Care* 7(1998): 98-102.

--- "Rationing Within the NHS Should Be Explicit: The Case For." *BMJ* 314 (1997): 1114-18.

--- "The Moral Importance of Informed Consent in Medical Research: Concluding Reflections." *Informed Consent in Medical Research*. Eds. L. Doyal and J. Tobias. London: BMJ Press, 2000. 309-17.

Doyal, L. and I. Gough. *A Theory of Human Need*. London: Macmillan, 1991.

Doyal, L. and R. Harris. *Empiricism, Explanation and Rationality: An Introduction to the Philosophy of the Social Sciences*. London: Routledge & Kegan Paul, 1986.

Draft Guidance for Industry: Source Animal, Product, Preclinical and Clinical Issues Concerning the Use of Xenotransplantation Products in Humans. Food & Drug Administration. Rockville, MD: U.S. Department of Health and Human Services, 2001.

"Draft Public Health Service Guideline on Infectious Disease Issues in Xenotransplantation." Department of Health and Human Services, Public Health Service. *Federal Register*, 23 Sept. 1996. 49919-32.

"Draft Report of the Infection Surveillance Steering Group of the UKXIRA." Official Stmt. *Bulletin of Medical Ethics* (1999): 9-11.

Dworkin, R. "Rights as Trumps." *Theories of Rights*. Ed. J. Waldron. Oxford: Oxford University Press, 1984. 153-67.

Dworkin, R. *Life's Dominion: An Argument About Abortion, Euthanasia and Individual Freedom*. New York: Vintage, 1994.

Dworkin, R. *Limits: The Role of the Law in Bioethical Decision Making*. Bloomington, IN: Indiana University Press, 1996.

"Emerging and other Communicable Diseases Surveillance and Control." *Report of WHO Consultation on Xenotransplantation*. WHO/EMC/ZOO/98.2. 28-30 October 1997. Geneva: World Health Organization.

"Emerging and other Communicable Diseases Surveillance and Control." *Xenotransplantation: Guidance on Infectious Disease Prevention and Management*. WHO/EMC/ZOO/98.2. 28-30 October 1997. Geneva: World Health Organization.

Engel, M. "Virginia Doctor Plans Company to Arrange Sale of Human Kidneys." *Washington Post*, 19 September 1983, A9.

Ethical and Policy Issues in Research Involving Human Participants. National Bioethics Advisory Commission. Washington, D.C., 2000.

"EU Road Accident Deaths Edge Lower in 1998." *Wall Street Journal Europe*, 7 July 2000, at 2.

European Network of Scientific Co-operation on Medicine and Human Rights. *The Human Rights, Ethical and Moral Dimensions of Health Care*. Strasbourg: Council of Europe.

"Europeans and Biotechnology in 2002." 2nd ed. 3 Dec. 2003. http://europa.eu.int/comm/public_opinion/archives/eb/ebs_177_en.pdf.

Evans, R.W. "Money Matters: Should Ability to Pay Ever be a Consideration in Gaining Access to Transplantation?" *Transplant. Proc*. 21 (1989): 3419-23.

--- "Understanding Xenophobia Induced by Economics." *Graft* 4 (2001): 154-56.

Evans, R.W. and D.L. Manninen. *Public Opinion Concerning Organ Donation, Procurement, and Distribution: Results of a National Probability Sample Survey*. Seattle: Battelle Human Affairs Research Centers, 1987.

Fano, Alix, et al. "Of Pigs, Primates and Plagues: A Layperson's Guide to the Problems with Animal-to-Human Organ Transplants." *Medical Research Modernization Committee, Campaign for Responsible Transplantation*. <http://www.crt-online.org/mrmc.html>

"FDA Proposed Rule Requires Public Access to Information on Gene Therapy, Xenotransplantation Clinical Trials." *Transplant News*, 16 Feb. 2001.

"Financing Health Services in Developing Countries." Washington, D.C.: The World Bank, 1987.

Fishman, A. *Fishman's Pulmonary Diseases and Disorders*. Vol. 1. New York: McGraw-Hill, 1998.

Fishman, J. "The Process of Discovery." *Bulletin of the World Health Organization* 77.1 (1999): 73-74.

--- "The Risk of Infection in Xenotransplantation." *Xenotransplantation: Scientific Frontiers and Public Policy*. Eds. J. Fishman et al. New York: Annals of the New York Academy of Sciences 862 (1998): 45-66.

Fox, J. "Blood Products Part of FDA Xenotransplant Plan." *Nature Biotechnology* 18 (March 2000): 258.

Fox, M. and J. McHale. "Xenotransplantation: The Ethical and Legal Ramifications." *Medical Law Review* 6 (1998): 42-61.

Fox, R. and J. Swazey. *Courage to Fail: A Social View of Organ Transplants and Dialysis*. Chicago: University of Chicago Press, 1974.

--- *Spare Parts: Organ Replacement in American Society*. New York: Oxford University Press, 1992.

Fox, R. *The Sociology of Medicine: A Participant Observer's View*. Englewood Cliffs, NJ: Prentice-Hall, 1989.

Fredrickson, D. "Asilomar and Recombinant DNA: The End of the Beginning." *Biomedical Politics*. Ed. K. Hanna. Washington, D.C.: National Academy Press, 1991. 258-98.

Fredrickson, J. "He's All Heart…And a Little Pig Too: A Look at the FDA Draft Xenotransplant Guidelines." *Food and Drug Law Journal* 52 (1997): 429-51.

Frey, R. "Moral Standing, the Value of Lives, and Speciesism." *Between the Species*. 4.3 (1988): 191-201.

--- *Interests and Rights: The Case Against Animals*. Oxford: Clarendon Press, 1980.

--- *Rights, Killing, & Suffering*. London: Basil Blackwell, 1983.

Friend, P. and B. Sohn. "Determining the Rate of Growth of a Pig Organ in a Primate." *Graft* 4 (2001): 111-14.

Furrow, B. *Bioethics: Health Care Law and Ethics*. 2nd ed. n.p. 1991.

Garrett, L. *The Coming Plague: Newly Emerging Diseases in a World Out of Balance*. New York: Farrar, Straus and Giroux, 1994.

Gay, C. "Open Your Wallets: All the Technology Means We'll be Spending Less on Health Care in the Years Ahead, Right? Fat Chance." *The Wall Street*, Journal 18 October 1999, R9.

Genethics. Eds. H. Bernard and C. Cookson. Basel: Ciba-Geigy, 1995.

Gewirth, A. "Are There Any Absolute Rights?" *Theories of Rights*. Ed. J. Waldron. Oxford: Oxford University Press, 1984. 91-109.

Giddens, A. *The Consequences of Modernity*. Cambridge: Polity Press, 1990.

Gilman, B. and S. Gejdenson. "Preventing Disease: We're All in This Together." *International Herald Tribune*, 4 July 2000, 6.

Glaberson, W. "Legal Pioneers Seek to Raise Lowly Status of Animals." *The New York Times*, 18 August 1999, 1.

Goodfield, J. *Playing God: Genetic Engineering and the Manipulation of Life*, Random House: New York, 1977.

Goodman, D. et al. "Preventing Acute Vascular Rejection." *Graft* 4 (2001): 47-51.

Gore, A. "Procurement and Allocation of Human Organs for Transplantation." *Hearings on H.R. 5580 Before the Subcommittee on Investigations and Oversight of the House Committee on Science and Technology*. 98th Cong., 1st Sess. 361, 1983.

Gray, J. "Nature Bites Back." *The Politics of Risk Society*. Ed. J. Franklin. Malden: Blackwell, 1998. 43-49.

Grigsby, B., ed. *1999 Report on U.S. Telemedicine Activity*. Association of Telehealth Service Providers: Washington, D.C., 2000.

Groth, C.G. and M.E. Breimer. "Xenotransplantation in Sweden." *Bulletin of the World Health Organization*. 77.1 (1999): 75-76.

Gruskin, S. and B. Tarantola. "Health and Human Rights." *The Oxford Textbook of Public Health*. Eds. Detels et al. 4th ed. Oxford: Oxford University Press, n.d.

Grygotis, M. "Mexican girl's death while waiting for a transplant in US sparks debate over foreign national transplant policy." *Transplant News*, 15 September 2000, 12.

Guidance on Making Proposals to Conduct Xenotransplantation on Human Subjects. British Ministry of Health. United Kingdom Xenotransplantation Interim Regulatory Authority, 1998.

H.R. Report No. 960. 101st Cong. 2nd sess. Part 1. Washington: GPO, 1990. 29.

Habermas, J. *Moral Consciousness and Communicative Action*. Trans. C. Lenhardt and S. Nicholsen. Cambridge, Mass: MIT Press, 1990.

--- *Between Facts and Norms: Contributions to a Discourse Theory of Law and Democracy*. Trans. W. Rehg. Cambridge, Mass.: MIT Press, 1996.

--- *Communication and the Evolution of Society*. Cambridge: MIT Press, 1989.

--- *Theory and Practice*. Boston: Beacon Press, 1973.

Hahn, R. "Ethical Issues." *Principles and Practice of Public Health Surveillance*. Eds. S. Teutsch and R. Churchill. New York: Oxford University Press, 1994. 175-89.

Hamsun, K. *Growth of the Soil*. Trans. W. Worster. New York: Vintage, 1972.

Haraway, D. *Simians, Cyborgs, and Women: The Reinvention of Nature*. New York: Routledge, 1991.

Harris, J. "QALYfying the Value of Life." *Journal of Medical Ethics* 13 (1987): 117-23.

--- *Kennedy Institute of Ethics Journal* (December 1999).

--- *The Value of Life: An Introduction to Medical Ethics*. London: Routledge, 1985.

--- "More and Better Justice." *Philosophy and Medical Welfare*. Eds. J. Bell and S. Mendus. Cambridge: Cambridge University Press, 1988.

--- "Must Doctors Save Their Patients." *Journal of Medical Ethics* 9 (1983): 211-18.

--- "The Ethics of National Ethics Committees." *Journal of the Royal College of Physicians of London* 28 (1994): 323-24.

--- *Clones, Genes, and Immortality: Ethics and the Genetic Revolution*. New York: Oxford University Press, 1998.

Harris, J. and S. Woods. "Rights and Responsibilities of Individuals Participating in Medical Research." *Informed Consent in Medical Research*. Eds. L. Doyal and J. Tobias. London: BMJ Books, 2001. 276-82.

Health and Human Rights. Eds. Mann, J., et al. New York: Routledge, 1999. 7-23.

Heaver, R. *Managing Primary Health Care: Implications of the Health Transition*. Washington, D.C.: The World Bank, 1995.

Heneine, W., et al. "Identification of a Human Population Infected with Simian Foamy Viruses." *Nature Medicine* 4.4 (1998): 403-07.

Henry J. Kaiser Family Foundation, "Medicaid and the Uninsured." *Kaiser Commission on Key Facts* (Jan. 2003).

Hoffenberg, R. "Should Organs From Patients in Permanent Vegetative States be Used for Transplantation?" *The Lancet* 350 (1997): 9087.

Hohfeld, W. *Fundamental Legal Conceptions As Applied in Judicial Reasoning*. 1919. New Haven, CT: Yale University Press, 1964.

Hooper, E. *The River: A Journey to the Source of HIV and AIDS*. Boston: Little, Brown & Co., 1999.

Hosenpud, J. et al. "The Registry of the International Society for Heart and Lung Transplantation: Seventeenth Official Report—2000." *The Journal of Heart and Lung Transplantation* 19 (2000): 909-31.

Howden-Chapman, P., J. Carter, J. and N. Woods. "Blood Money: Blood Donors' Attitudes to Changes in the New Zealand Blood Transfusion Service." *British Medical Journal* 312 (1996): 1131-32.

<http://cnn.com/HEALTH/9909/30/health.transplants.reut/index.html>.

Hubbard, R. *The Politics of Women's Biology*. New Brunswick, NJ: Rutgers University Press, 1990.

"Huge Disparity Between Americans on Transplant Waiting List, Number Who Donate Sparks Action." *Transplant News*, 16 March 2001.

Hugo, V. *Les Miserables*.Trans. L. Fahnestock. New York: Signet Classic, 1987.

Hume, D. *A Treatise of Human Nature*. 1740. London: J.M. Dent, 1911.

Ignatieff, M. *The Needs of Strangers*. New York: Viking Penguin, 1984.

Institute of Medicine. *Antimicrobial Resistance: Issues and Options*. Forum on Emerging Infections. Washington, D.C.: National Academy Press, 1998.

Institute of Medicine. *Xenotransplantation: Science, Ethics and Public Policy*. Washington, D.C.: National Academy Press, 1996.

International Society for Heart and Lung Transplantation Issues. Comprehensive Guidelines on How and When to Proceed with Animal-to-Human Heart and Lung Transplants. ISHLT Press Release. Dallas, TX. 15 Dec. 2000, 1-4.

International Telecommunications Satellite Organization (Intelsat) Agreement with Annexes. *Treaties in Active Service*. 18 United States Treaties 2410 (1971): 6347.

Jacobs, L. *Rights and Deprivation*. Oxford: Clarendon Press, 1993.

Jacobs, P. *The Economics of Health and Medical Care*. 4th ed. Gaithersburg, MD: Aspen Publishers, 1997.

Jacobson v. Massachusetts 197 US 11, 25-27 (1905).

Johnson, K. "Organ Procurement Organizations." *Organ Procurement, Preservation and Distribution in Transplantation*. Ed. M. Phillips. Richmond, VA: UNOS, 1996.

Jones, J. et al. "Successful Hand Transplantation." *The New England Journal of Medicine* 17 Aug. 2000, 468-73.

Kaiser, L. and F.G. Hayden "Hospitalizing Influenza in Adults." *Current Clinical Topics in Infectious Diseases*. 19 (1999): 112.

Kant, I. *Lectures on Ethics*. Trans. L. Infield. Indianapolis, IN: Hackett, 1979.

Kanter, R. *Commitment and Community: Communes and Utopias in Sociological Perspective*. Cambridge: Mass.: Harvard University Press, 1972.

Kennedy, I. *Animal Tissues into Humans*. Advisory Group on the Ethics of Xenotransplantation. London: Stationery Office, 1997.

Kennedy, I. "The Case for Presumed Consent in Organ Donation." *The Lancet*. (1998): 351: 9116.

Kennedy, I. and A. Grubb. *Medical Law*. 3rd ed. London: Butterworths, 2000.

Keon, W. "Heart Transplantation in Perspective." *Journal of Cardiological Surgery*. 14 (1999): 147-51.

Kevles, D. *In the Name of Eugenics*. Berkeley: University of California Press, 1986.

Klotzko, A. "Pork Progress." *Scientific American*. November 1999: 48.

Kootstra, G. et al. "Twenty Percent More Kidneys Through a Non-Heartbeating Program." *Transplant. Proc.*, 23 (1991): 910.

Korsgren, O., et al. "Xenotransplanting Pancreatic Islets." *Graft* 4 (2001): 115-17.

Kumar, S. "India 'Xenotransplant' Doctors Granted Bail." *The Lancet* 349 (1997): 628.

Langer, R. and J. Vacanti. "Artificial Organs." *Scientific American*, September 1995: 130-133.

Leahy, M. *Against Liberation: Putting Animals in Perspective*. 1991. London: Routledge, 1994.

Leary, V. "The Right to Health in International Human Rights Law." *Health and Human Rights* 1 (1994): 25-56.

--- "Defining the Right to Health Care." *Health Care Reform: A Human Rights Approach*. Ed. A. Chapman. Washington, D.C.: Georgetown University Press, 1994. 87-105.

Lederberg, J. "Infectious History." *Science*. 288 (2000): 287-93.

Lenski, R. "The Cost of Antibiotic Resistance – From the Perspective of a Bacterium." *Antibiotic Resistance: Origins, Evolution, Selection and Spread*. New York: John Wiley & Sons, 1997. 131-51.

Levy, S. *The Antibiotic Paradox: How Miracle Drugs Are Destroying the Miracle*. New York: Plenum, 1992.

Linzey, A. "For Animal Rights." *The Liberation Debate: Rights At Issue*. Eds. M. Leahy and D. Cohn-Sherbok. London: Routledge, 1996.

Lundin, S. "Understanding Cultural Perspectives on Clinical Xenotransplantation." *Graft* 4 (2001): 150-53.

Lysaght, M. and P. Aebischer. "Encapsulated Cells as Therapy." *Scientific American* Apr.: 76-80.

Mahler, H. "The Challenge of Global Health: How Can We Do Better?" *Health and Human Rights* 2 (1994): 71-75.

"Man Who Received Baboon Liver in 1992 Became Infected With Baboon CMV." *Transplant News*, 14 October 1999.

Managed Care Systems and Emerging Infections: Challenges and Opportunities for Strengthening Surveillance, Research, and Prevention. Ed. J. Davis. Washington, D.C.: Institute of Medicine Forum on Emerging Infections, National Academy Press, 2000.

Mann, J. "Medicine and Public Health, Ethics and Human Rights." *Health and Human Rights*. Eds. Mann, J., et al. New York: Routledge, 1999. 439-52.

Mann, J. et al. "Health and Human Rights." *Health and Human Rights* 1 (1994): 7-23.

Massaquoi, H. *Destined to Witness: Growing Up Black in Nazi Germany*. New York: William Morrow, 1999.

Matthews, G. and R. Churchill. "Public Health Surveillance and the Law". *Principles and Practice of Public Health Surveillance*. Eds. S. Teutsch and R. Churchill. New York: Oxford University Press, 1994. 190-99.

Mauss, M. *The Gift*. London: Routledge, 1990.

McCarthy, T. *Ideals and Illusions: On Reconstruction and Deconstruction in Contemporary Critical Theory*. Cambridge: MIT Press, 1993.

McDougal, M., H. Lasswell and I. Vlasic. *Law and Public Order in Space*. New Haven, CT: Yale University Press, 1963.

McMullen, L. "Equitable Allocation of Human Organs: An Examination of the New Federal Regulation." *Journal of Legal Medicine* 20 (1999): 405-24.

Meslin, F., et. al. (1998), "Monitoring Infectious Diseases." *Xenotransplantation: Scientific Frontiers and Public Policy*. Eds. J. Fishman, D. Sachs and R. Shaikh. Vol. 862. New York: Annals of the New York Academy of Sciences, 1998. 205-10.

Michaels, M. "Determining the Risks of Xenozoonoses." *Graft* 4 (2001): 129-30.

Midgley, M. *Beast and Man: The Roots of Human Nature*. Ithaca, NY: Cornell University Press, 1978.

Miller, H. and G. Conko. "The Protocol's Illusionary Principle." *Nature Biotechnology,* 18 (2000): 360.

Moatti, J. "Researcher-Driven Versus Policy-Driven Economic Appraisal." *Xenotransplantation: Scientific Frontiers and Public Policy*. Eds. J. Fishman, D. Sachs and R. Shaikh. Vol. 862. New York: Annals of the New York Academy of Sciences, 1998. 188-201.

Nussbaum, M. "Human Capabilities, Female Human Beings." Eds. M. Nussbaum and J. Glover. *Women, Culture & Development: A Study of Human Capabilities*. Oxford: Clarendon, 1995. 61-104.

Onishi, A. et al. "Pig Cloning by Microinjection of Fetal Fibroblast Nuclei." *Science* 289 (2000): 1188.

"Organ Procurement Organizations: Alternatives Being Developed to More Accurately Assess Performance." *Report to the Ranking Minority Member, Committee on Labor and Human Resources, U.S. Senate.* Washington, D.C.: GAO, 1997.

Orlans, F. and T. Beauchamp et al. *The Human Use of Animals: Case Studies in Ethical Choice*. New York: Oxford University Press, 1998.

Orwell, G. *Homage to Catalonia: Looking Back on the Spanish War*. Harmondsworth: Penguin, 1968.

Otten, M. "Surveillance Issues in Developing Countries." *Principles and Practice of Public Health Surveillance*. Eds. S. Teutsch and R. Churchill. New York: Oxford University Press, 1994. 235-55.

Patience, C. "Determining and Preventing the Potential PERV Problem." *Graft* 4 (2001): 133-34.

Patience C., Y. Takeuchi, and R.A. Weiss. "Infection of Human Cells By an Endogenous Retrovirus of Pigs." *Nature Medicine* 3 (1997): 282-86.

Pecoul, B. et al. "Access to Essential Drugs in Poor Countries: A Lost Battle?" *JAMA* 281 (1999): 361-67.

"Penicillin's Finder Assays Its Future." *New York Times*, 26 June 1945, 21.

Persing, D.H. "Xenotransplantation and Infectious Diseases." *Xenotransplantation: The Transplantation of Organs and Tissues Between Species*. Ed. D.K.C. Cooper. 2nd ed. Berlin: Springer, 1997. 749-65.

"PERV data renew xeno debate." *Nature Biotechnology* 18 (2000): 1032-33.

Peters, D. et al. "Health Expenditures, Services and Outcomes in Africa: Basic Data and Cross-National Comparisons 1990-1996." *The World Bank Health, Nutrition and Population Publication Series*. Washington, D.C.: World Bank, 1999.

Pierce, G. "UNOS History." *Organ Procurement, Preservation and Distribution in Transplantation*. Ed. M. Phillips. Richmond, VA: UNOS, 1996.

Piercy, M. *Woman on the Edge of Time*. New York: Fawcett Crest, 1976.

Pierson, R. and G. Miller. "Late Graft Failure: Lessons from Clinical Experimental Thoracic Organ Transplantation." *Graft* 3 (2000): 88-92.

Pinel, J. *Essential Drugs: Practical Guidelines*. Fevrier: Medicins San Frontières, 1993.

Platt, J. and S. Lin. "The Future Promises of Xenotransplantation." *Xenotransplantation: Scientific Frontiers and Public Policy*. Eds. J. Fishman, D. Sachs and R. Shaikh. Vol. 862. New York: Annals of the New York Academy of Sciences, 1998. 5-18.

"Poll reveals backing for xenotransplants." Nature 391 (1998): 315.

Porter, R. *The Greatest Benefit to Mankind: A Medical History of Humanity*. New York: Norton & Company, 1997.

Potter, V. *Bioethics: Bridge to the Future*. Englewood Cliffs, NJ: Prentice-Hall, 1971.

Powers, A., et al. "Permeability Assessment of Capsules for Islet Transplantation." *Bioartificial Organs: Science, Medicine and Technology*. Ed. A. Prokop et al. New York: New York Academy of Sciences, 1997. 208-16

Presnall, J. *Artificial Organs*. Lucent: San Diego, 1997.

Price, D. "Organ Transplant Initiatives: The Twilight Zone." *Journal of Medical Ethics* 23 (1997): 170-75.

Proctor, R. *Racial Hygiene*. Cambridge: Harvard University Press, 1988.

Prusiner, S. "The Prion Diseases." *Scientific American*, Jan. 1995.

Rawls, J. *A Theory of Justice*. 1971. Cambridge, Mass.: Harvard University Press, 1999.

Rawls, J. et al. *Liberty, Equality and the Law*. Cambridge: Cambridge University Press, 1987.

Regan, T. *The Case for Animal Rights*. Berkeley: University of California Press, 1983.

Renteln, A. *International Human Rights: Universalism Versus Relativism*. Sage: London, 1990.

"Report of the Extraordinary Meeting of the Conference of the Parties For the Adoption of the Protocol on Biosafety to the Convention on Biological Diversity." *Convention on Biological Diversity*. United Nations Document UNEP/CBD/ExCOP/1/3, 20 February 2000.

Rescher, N. Risk: *A Philosophical Introduction to the Theory of Risk Evaluation and Management*. Lanham: University Press of America, 1983.

Reubinoff, B. et al. "Embryonic Stem Cell Lines from Human Blastocysts: Somatic Differentiation in Vitro." *Nature Biotechnology* 18 (2000): 399-405.

Richards, J. "Nephrarious Goings On: Kidney Sales and Moral Arguments." *Journal of Medical Philosophy*. 21 (1996): 375-416.

Richards, J. and A.S. Daar. "The Case for Allowing Kidney Sales." *The Lancet* 351 (1998): 1950-52.

Rivard, M. "Toward a General Theory of Constitutional Personhood: A Theory of Constitutional Personhood for Transgenic Humanoid Species." *UCLA Law Review* 39 (1992): 1425.

Rivero, A. and T. Galan. "An International View of Patients' Rights, in European Network of Scientific Co-operation on Medicine and Human Rights." *The Human Rights, Ethical and Moral Dimensions of Health Care*. Strasbourg: Council of Europe, 1998. 101-09.

Rogers, A. and D. de Bousingen. *Bioethics in Europe*. Strasbourg: Council of Europe Press, 1995.

Rogers, L. "Transplant Pioneer Plans to Offer Pig Hearts in Britain." *The Sunday Times*, 31 October 1999, 7.

Rothfeder, J. *Heart Rhythms*. Little Brown: Boston. n.d.

Rowland, R. "Doctors Look for Liver Transplant Alternatives." 3 October 1999. <http://www.cnn.com>.

Rubinstein, D. *Marx and Wittgenstein: Social Praxis and Social Explanation*. London: Routledge & Kegan Paul, 1981.

Rudacille, D. *The Scalpel and the Butterfly: The War Between Animal Research and Animal Protection*. New York: Farrar, Strauss & Giroux, 2000.

Scott, R. "The Terrible Imbalance: Human Organs and Tissues for Therapy – A Review of Demand and Supply." *Journal of Contemporary Health Law and Policy*. 9 (1993): 139-58.

Sen, A. "Capability and Well-Being." *The Quality of Life*. Eds. M. Nussbaum and A. Sen. Oxford: Clarendon Press, 1993. 30-53.

Shannon, T. *An Introduction to Bioethics*. 3rd ed. New York: Paulist Press, 1979.

Singer, P. *Animal Liberation*. 1975. Wellingborough: Thorsons, 1983.

--- *Practical Ethics*. Cambridge: Cambridge University Press, 1979.

Smart, J.J.C. and B. Williams. *Utilitarianism For and Against*. Cambridge: University Press, 1973.

Smith, G. *Human Rights and Biomedicine*. The Hague: Kluwer Law International, 2000.

Smith, W. "Is Bioethics Ethical?" *The Weekly Standard*, 3 April 2000, 26-30.

Squinto, S. and W. Fodor. "Engineering of Xenografts to Provide Organs for Human Transplantation." *Xenotransplantation: The Transplantation of Organs and Tissues Between Species*. Ed. D.K.C. Cooper. 2nd ed. Berlin: Springer, 1997. 659-64.

Stapleton, Stephanie. "HHS Wants to Change How Organs are Allocated for Transplant." *American Medical News*, 16 March 1998, 11-12.

Stolberg, S. "Patients' Lives on the Line in Battle over Transplants." *New York Times*, 25 March 1998, A1.

Stoye, J. et al. "Endogenous Retroviruses: A Potential Problem for Xenotransplantation." *Xenotransplantation: Scientific Frontiers and Public Policy*. Eds. J. Fishman, D. Sachs and R. Shaikh. Vol. 862. New York: Annals of the New York Academy of Sciences, 1998. 67-74.

Swindle, M. "Defining Appropriate Health Status and Management Programs for Specific-Pathogen-Free Swine for Xenotransplantation." *Xenotransplantation: Scientific Frontiers and Public Policy*. Eds. J. Fishman, D. Sachs and R. Shaikh. Vol. 862. New York: Annals of the New York Academy of Sciences, 1998. 111-20.

Taniguchi, S. and D.K.C Cooper. "Clinical Xenotransplantation – A Brief Review of the World Experience." *Xenotransplantation: The Transplantation of Organs and Tissues Between Species*. Ed. D.K.C. Cooper. 2nd ed. Berlin: Springer, 1997. 778-79.

The World Health Report 1999: Making a Difference. Geneva: World Health Organization, 1999.

The World Health Report 2000: Health Systems: Improving Performance. Geneva: World Health Organization, 2000.

Third Annual Report, September 1999 – November 2000. British Ministry of Health. United Kingdom Xenotransplantation Interim Regulatory Authority, 2000.

Tibell, A. "Regulating Clinical Xenotransplantation in Europe." *Graft* 4 (2001): 157-59.

Titmuss, R. *The Gift Relationship: From Human Blood to Social Policy*. New York: New Press, 1997.

Touraine, A. "Society as Utopia." *Utopia: The Search for the Ideal Society in the Western World*. Ed. R. Schaer. New York: Oxford University Press, 2000. 18-30.

"Transgenic Pigs." *Nature Biotechnology* 18 (2000): 365.

Transplant News, 14 May 2000, 1-2.

Turville-Heitz, M. "Violent Opposition." *Scientific American*, February 2000: 32-34.

Ubel, P. *Pricing Life: Why It's Time for Health Care Rationing*. Cambridge: MIT Press, 2000.

UK Donor Identity Plan Aims to Double Size of National Donor Registry." *Transplant News*, 30 March 2001, 7.

United Nations General Assembly Resolution 217 (III). 10 December 10 1948, art. 25, 27 and 22.

7 US Code. Sec. 2143. 1999.

Utopia: The Search for the Ideal Society in the Western World. Ed. R. Schaer. New York: Oxford University Press, 2000.

Van Rongen, E. "The View of the Health Council of the Netherlands." *Bulletin of the World Health Organization*. 77.1 (1999): 79-81.

Vanderpool, H. "Commentary: A Critique of Clark's Frightening Xenotransplantation Scenario." *The Journal of Law, Medicine & Ethics* 27 (1999): 153-57.

---. "Overcoming the Risks of 'Ethical Rejection." *Graft* 4 (2001): 140-42.

Vanhove, B., J. Renard and J. Soulillou. "Genetic Engineering in the Pig." *Xenotransplantation: Scientific Frontiers and Public Policy*. Eds. J. Fishman, D. Sachs and R. Shaikh. Vol. 862. New York: Annals of the New York Academy of Sciences, 1998. 28-36.

Vincent, R. *Human Rights and International Relations*. Cambridge: University Press, 1997.

Wainwright, M. *Miracle Cure: The Story of Antibiotics*. Oxford: Blackwell, 1990. *Wall Street Journal*, 22 September 1999, A15.

Watanabe, T. "Infectious Drug Resistance." *Scientific American* 217 (1967): 19-27.

Weaver, G. and A. Williams. "A Mother's Gift: The Milk of Human Kindness." *The Gift Relationship: From Human Blood to Social Policy*. Eds. A. Oakley and J. Ashton. New York: New Press, 1997. 319-32.

Weijer, C. "The Ethical Analysis of Risk." *Journal of Law, Medicine & Ethics*. 28 (2000): 344-61.

Weiss, R., S. Magre, and Y. Takeuchi. "Infection Hazards of Xenotransplantation." *Journal of Infection*. 40 (2000): 21-25.

Wells, M. "Overview of FDA Regulation of Human Cellular and Tissue-Based Products." *Food and Law Journal*. 52 (1997): 401-08.

Whitehead, A. "Rejecting Organs: The Organ Allocation Process and the Americans with Disabilities Act." *American Journal of Law and Medicine*. 24(1996): 481-97.

Williams, G., J. Popay, and P. Bissell. "Public Health Risks in the Material World: Barriers to Social Movements in Health." *Medicine, Health and Risk: Sociological Approaches*. Ed. J. Gabe. Oxford: Blackwell, 1995. 113-32.

Witte, W. "Impact of Antibiotic Use in Animal Feeding on Resistance of Bacterial Pathogens in Humans." *Antibiotic Resistance: Origins, Evolution, Selection and Spread*. New York: John Wiley and Sons, 1997. 61-75.

Wittgenstein, L. *Philosophical Investigations*. 3rd ed. Trans. G. Anscombe. 1953. New York: Macmillan, 1958.

"World's First Double-Hand Transplant Showing Improvement." *Transplant News*, 29 Feb. 2000, 5.

"World's First Internal Transplant of a Miniature LVAD Performed at Texas Heart Institute." *Transplant News*, 28 April 2000, 7.

Xenotransplantation Subcommittee of the Biological Response Modifiers Advisory Committee. Food & Drug Administration. Washington, D.C.: Beta Reporting, 2000.

Xenotransplantation: International Policy Issues. Paris: OECD Publications, 1999.

Young, N. "This Little Piggy Saved Stroke Victim Maribeth." *The Express*, 4 October 1999, 15.

Index

Credits

p.4 *We offer excellent medical coverage but the policy does not cover pre-existing organs.*
Reprinted with permission from the artist, Aaron Bacall, Staten Island, New York, abacall@msn.com.

p.39 *Unfortunately, Carolyn, your body has rejected your face lift.*
CLOSE TO HOME © John McPherson. Reprinted with permission of UNIVERSAL PRESS SYNDICATE. All Rights Reserved.

p.79 *We are comforted by the knowledge that at twenty-six years of age, he had lived a long and full life.*
© 2003 Frank Cotham from cartoonbank.com. All Rights Reserved.

p.101 *This patient has a rare form of medical insurance.*
© The New Yorker Collection 1994 Frank Cotham from cartoonbank.com. All Rights Reserved.

p.115 *Don't forget to take a handful of our complimentary antibiotics on your way out.*
© The New Yorker Collection 1998 Mick Stevens from cartoonbank.com. All Rights Reserved.

p.132 *So Doctor, how is your gene splicing research going?*
© 1993 Norman Dog.